THE BODY IS THE HERO

THE BODY IS THE HERO

BY *Ronald J. Glasser, M.D.*

RANDOM HOUSE

New York

Library of Congress Cataloging in Publication Data

Glasser, Ronald J
The body is the hero.

1. Immunology. I. Title.
QR181.7.G58   616.07'9   75-40568
ISBN 0-394-40013-5

Manufactured in the United States of America

2 4 6 8 9 7 5 3

FIRST EDITION

CONTENTS

1. A Terrifying Experiment of Nature   3
2. In the Beginning   18
3. Forerunners: The First Insights   29
4. Jenner and Pasteur   47
5. Our Immune System: Early Discoveries   59
6. Our Immune System: The Protectors   68
7. Our Immune System: The Killers   82
8. Our Immune System: The Mastermind   90
9. Rh Incompatibility: The Riddle   100
10. The Riddle Solved   112
11. Immunization: Why It Works   126
12. Immunization: How It Works   147
13. Mistakes of Nature   163
14. The Body Against Itself   182
15. Rejection: The Battle of Transplants   194
16. Cancer   206
17. Beyond Immunology   226

THE BODY
IS THE HERO

I

A Terrifying
Experiment of Nature

DESPITE OUR CULTURE and its abhorrence of death there are some deaths that are welcome, even those of children. There are diseases where the illness is so grim, the pain and suffering so bitter and constant that even with our own fears of loss and loneliness, our own terror of the unknown, death does not seem so frightening, nor when it comes, such a horrible burden. Combined immunodeficiency is one of these illnesses. It is a disease afflicting infants born seemingly perfect but without the chemical inheritance of a billion years floating in their bloodstream—children doomed, in truth, from the day they are born. So grotesque is their dying that everyone, parents, neighbors, doctors, nurses, friends, all welcome their death, wondering why these children were ever born at all.

We exist today, we have survived to the present, because in the long struggle of evolution there began to develop in our ancestors and then within each of us a system of protection so sophisticated and so powerful that after a billion years of continuous battle, despite all the ruptured appendices, broken

[3]

bones, burns, pneumonias and meningitises, we have prevailed and been permitted to go on.

From the beginnings of life it has been the thousands of single-cell microbes—always there trying to destroy us everywhere along our way—more than any cataclysm of nature, that have been our real opponents in the long struggle for existence. Our survival throughout evolution individually and as a species has rested on the weapons our bodies have developed to meet their relentless, unending attacks.

Nowhere can the desperateness of this struggle, nor the implication of how dependent we are on our defenses, be more graphically seen than in the case of children born without the ability to protect themselves from these microbes. In every generation there are those who come into being perfect in every way except one—the ability to mount an immune defense. If we were born without this evolutionary heritage, their fate would be ours, their brief history that of our whole race.

In the early days of vaccination, the smallpox virus was scratched onto the arm or foot of an infant in the first month of life. But something was wrong. At medical meetings and in correspondences, physicians talked to one another of the occasional healthy child who had been vaccinated and then gone on to die within two weeks. It was a rare occurrence, but the isolated reports began to add up, and a feeling gradually developed among the various medical societies that deaths from smallpox vaccination were somehow related to the early age of the patients. Adults who were vaccinated did not die; they may have become ill, may have had fever, but they did not die. To protect the children, the societies recommended that vaccinations be given at three months of age, but still some children died. Then the recommendation was extended to six months, then nine months.

There had always been minor complications resulting from vaccination—rashes, fever, an occasional seizure—but it was felt the benefits far outweighed the few risks. For centuries smallpox had ravaged the world. An immunized population able to check the smallpox virus was considered worth the price when balanced against the small percentage of children affected by what were in general relatively minor complications.

But the fact could not be ignored that occasionally a totally healthy infant would be immunized and within two weeks be dead. In these children the vaccination sore did not, as was expected, simply come to a head, crust over and drop off. Instead it spread quickly over the whole arm. Within two days the single pustle had become a hundred, within a week the child's arm was nothing but an open, weeping sore. Eventually his eyes and his mouth became involved, then his ears. He began coughing up blood and having bloody diarrhea. The sores spread. Horrified, their fear giving way to desperation and desperation to terror, the parents watched helplessly while each day their child was consumed before their very eyes.

This tragedy may have been limited to a very few children, but it was so unexpected, so devastating and so universally fatal that physicians, without knowing what it was that caused this bizarre and terrifying complication, tried the only thing they could—to buy time by postponing the vaccination itself. But still the deaths did not stop. Even with the delayed vaccinations, children still died and in the same numbers. It seemed as if those who died were doomed from the beginning, that those who would have died when vaccinated at three months died instead when they were vaccinated at six months, while those who were not vaccinated at six months died when they were vaccinated at nine.

However, postponing the time of vaccination did have one positive result; it gave physicians the opportunity to make an important observation: those children who died after being vaccinated toward the end of their first year of life seemed to have suffered from a much higher incidence of colds, ear infections, tonsillitises and pneumonias than other children of the same age. Some literally had one cold after another from almost the time of their birth until their death.

It was a crucial, clinical observation, and the members of the American Academy of Pediatrics finally acted on it, recommending, without even being sure why, the further and final delay in smallpox vaccination until one year of age, so that those children who were susceptible to recurrent infections could be identified and not be vaccinated at all. So stringent was this recommendation, so disastrous a failure to comply that today there is no board-certified pediatrician in the United States who

[5]

ignores it. What the members of the Academy did not know was why those children who had one infection after another would be dead within two weeks of being given a vaccine that was virtually harmless to anyone else.

Today we realize that the children who died were those born without any immune defense, and in fact all that was gained by halting their vaccination was a little time, and not very good time at that. Instead of a dramatic, quick death resulting from the pox virus scratched on their arms, these children would go on to be slowly, relentlessly destroyed by infections, by the millions of microbes, the bacteria, viruses and fungi that surround us, slowly eaten away until by the age of two or three they would be dead anyway.

AT ABOUT TWO MONTHS of age the average infant begins to have between six to eight colds a year. These upper-respiratory infections are usually short-lived affairs—a few days of runny nose, crankiness, a little diarrhea, and the baby's well again. The virus has been neutralized by the first part of the child's immune system—the white cells circulating throughout his bloodstream—and by the second part of his immune defense, antibodies—proteins his body makes with no other function than to seek out and attack bacteria and viruses. Not only is each cold virus summarily destroyed but his body is primed, in case the same virus comes back, to destroy it, this time even before it has gained a foothold, before it can cause him a single sniffle or cough.

The viral attacks, however, continue. A few weeks or a few days later a new virus gets into the baby's nose or throat. There are another two or three days of fever, the same crankiness and stuffiness that were there before, until his body can process the new attacking organism, make the appropriate antibodies and send in the right number of white cells to destroy it. It is a series of events—microbial attack, counterattack, antibody production, viral neutralization and destruction—as rhythmical as life itself.

But for the unfortunate child born without an immune system, there is no rhythm. The viruses are not neutralized, nor are they destroyed. They continue to grow and multiply. The dry hacking coughs go on and on, the fevers persist, the restlessness continues. What every parent is sure will pass does not. The cough and the restlessness continue, the cold does not resolve, the runny nose does not stop.

THE FIRST VAGUE FEAR that something may be wrong with their baby begins to stir within the new parents. With his very first sniffle they had taken their child to the pediatrician and had been assured that it was nothing more than a simple cold, told to use a mist tent or perhaps given a prescription for a mild decongestant. But the baby's nose stays stuffed, and not being able to breathe properly, he begins having trouble feeding. Without asking the doctor, the parents may double the dose of the decongestant, turn up the mist in the tent even higher, or perhaps use a home remedy or a drug that had worked on their neighbor's child. Yet their baby continues to fret.

They fight their growing suspicion. After all, the child had been well before this cold—absolutely normal since birth. What they don't know is that during those early months of normalcy their infant, like any other newborn, was protected from the viruses and bacteria in the air he breathed, in the water he drank and in the food he ate by preformed antibodies transferred from his mother. These were antibodies that her body had already made to protect her, that were already in her circulation, and just before birth had entered her baby's bloodstream to protect him at delivery and for a short time after. Like any protein, they eventually break down, and if the newborn has no ability to make his own, he will be left unprotected within a few months of birth.

There are different classes of antibodies, distinguished one from the other by their different physical and chemical properties. They are made up of the proteins which survived the chemical evolution that preceded life. The smallest of these antibodies, those the scientists call IgG (gamma globulin), are small enough to cross the placenta and are able to accumulate in the infant's circulation. So great is this transfer mechanism that at birth newborns have more IgG's in their own circulation than their mothers have in theirs. The antibodies transferred from the mother are the infant's only defense against the teeming world he faces the moment he is born. But antibodies don't last forever in anyone. Gradually decaying as they move through our bodies, breaking up, fractionating, the maternal antibodies are destroyed by the infant's own circulation and organs by the end of six to eight weeks. But they have fulfilled their function, have given the newborn the time he needs for his own immune system, which has been gearing up since birth, to take over the production of his own antibodies, protecting him as he was protected by his mother.

It takes time for the chemistry of immunology to begin to work, for the child's immune system to process the new attackers, to learn what it has to do. But the immunodeficient child cannot make his own antibodies. As his mother's antibodies gradually disappear from his bloodstream, he is left unprotected, at the mercy of organisms a trillionth his size. These organisms keep attacking, and like pieces of shrapnel, eventually cut him down. The colds are only the beginning, the opening skirmishes in a war without quarter, without mercy and without hope, a war first begun a billion years before, in the original primeval seas.

When the first cold does not resolve, when in a few days their baby is not the least bit better, the parents take him back to the pediatrician. Again the doctor finds nothing unusual—infected tonsils, a little fluid in the middle ear and a stuffy nose, a slight wheezing in the lungs, but nothing more. The child actually looks healthy. The doctor may change the decongestant, add an expectorant, explain the use of Tylenol, or baby aspirin, but again he says, with conviction, that it is just a cold. He might even imply that the parents are being a bit overprotective, that this is their first child, and if they will learn to be patient, the cold will pass.

Yet it doesn't; the child does not get better. Still unable to breathe properly because of his stuffy nose, he cannot feed as he should, he begins to lose weight, or at any rate to stop gaining. The parents, unable to sleep because of their baby's fussiness, begin staying up with him. And he does not look quite the same any more. There is an apprehension in his face, a tension which is revealed even when he sleeps. He always looks a bit uncomfortable, or so it seems to his mother, who has watched him since birth. When she calls the doctor again, he asks if there is any change, and when she has to admit no, not really, he tells her to continue the same medications.

With a few more calls, if the baby is still coughing, is still not well, and if the mother is determined or distressed enough, the pediatrician may agree to see the child, but again he can find no outward change. The physical examination is the same as before: boggy and swollen mucous membranes, perhaps a little more throat inflammation than the previous visit, a little more fluid in the ears, but still really nothing greater than the normal reaction of tissues to a mild viral invasion. To placate the parents, the doctor may even take a chest film. It is absolutely negative, the lung fields are completely clear. Once more he consoles the mother, telling her it is just the flu, that it will pass. And he believes it.

Yet a physician must pay scrupulous attention to details, and the details on the chest film were not quite right. If he had looked closely at the X-ray, not just at the lung fields to see if there was a pneumonia, but at the other chest structures, he would have seen that above the heart there was no thymic shadow, that the thymus, a tiny organ normally in the chest of every infant, simply was not there. All he did was look at the lungs for pneumonia and there was none.

If good medicine implies the closest attention to details, it can be set to check itself (control its mistakes) simply by watchful waiting, and in the case of this child, even though the lack of the thymus was missed, watching became the appropriate treatment. Because in fact the pediatrician was right; the child was simply not ill enough for him to do more. At least not yet. There was no reason for a blood culture, or for a spinal tap, no reason for a urine culture. The child was not that ill. There was no apparent danger, no immediate emergency. Indeed, there was really still nothing to treat. It was even possible that the child might improve that the parents might finally be able to laugh away at least part of their fears.

There have been approximately a hundred rhino viruses detected which cause flu-like upper-respiratory symptoms. These viruses are all a bit different, having slightly different protein coverings, different internal proteins and different predispositions for various parts of the body. Some like the nose and grow there; others prefer the inner ear; still others, because of their own evolution, the pharynx or tonsils. The rhino viruses cause mild disease. They are not as destructive as other viruses;

they do not cause great tissue damage, nor do they spread as quickly to the deeper organs as do the herpes, smallpox or encephalitic viruses. In the world of viral organisms, which is as diverse as the animal kingdom itself, they are the least destructive. If the child is lucky enough to have been affected by one of these mild viruses rather than a more deadly one, it is possible that his illness may after a time subside on its own, or the virus simply reach a balance with his body where it lies dormant, waiting in a kind of blind stand-off in which neither the child nor the virus wins or loses.

But in this case any relief, whatever it may be and for whatever cause, is only temporary. Within a few more days the baby is obviously sicker. It has been almost two and a half weeks now since he first became ill, and the exhausted parents, anxious and confused, call the pediatrician again. There is no way of his comforting either of the parents now. They have talked with other families, friends, with aunts and uncles and grandmothers, and they know that normal colds do not hang on like this. They realize that something is wrong, and angrily they confront the doctor, expecting medicine to live up to its claims. Feeling abused himself, the pediatrician may in desperation, to placate the parents or because of his own growing suspicion that this child is not quite right, admit the infant to the hospital.

It is only on his rounds the next morning that he notices some white spots in the baby's mouth. The mother had noticed them herself for almost a week, but dismissed them as congealed milk or pieces of cereal and had not mention them to the doctor. But he knows they are not food and cannot be removed. Nor are they white, as the mother thought, but an off-shade of gray; they are a fungus growing in the child's mouth. It is not just a cold any more.

The mother senses the change in the doctor's tone, in his now definitive questions. "Has anybody in your family ever had a lot of infections?" he asks. "Have there been any deaths in your family during infancy or the newborn period? Any trouble with boils or abscesses and recurrent infections?" The questions have the chilling tone that has always been a part of medicine. "Anyone been ill after any of their vaccinations, or run long fevers, or had to be hospitalized? How long has he had these spots in his mouth?"

It is not a virus this time, but another type of attacker, a mold called *Candida albicans* that will grow on any warm, moist surface, on a piece of rotting bread, or if it can, in a newborn's warm, moist mouth. The reason the fungus attacks infants and not adults is that it cannot get a foothold in grown-ups. Adults have the antibodies to destroy it before it can grow, but they are not the kind of antibodies that cross the placenta, so for a time all newborns, even healthy ones, are indeed vulnerable. With no antibodies in the circulation to fight off the fungus, it begins to grow in their mouths, on the linings of their tongues and cheeks. But while the fungus grows, the normal infant's immune system processes it, makes the necessary antibodies and then, sending the antibodies to the site of infection, kills the fungus before it spreads too far.

Every pediatrician will, in the course of a year, see ten or fifteen infants with these grayish plaques growing in their mouth. The popular term for this condition is "thrush," and in most cases, despite its prevalence, it is a mild condition controlled by the infant himself. If too severe, it can be controlled by medications until the child's own immune system can come into play. Like all antibiotics, these anti-fungal medications only buy time. Penicillin, gentomycin, streptomycin, mycostatin are only tactical tools. They hold organisms in check, they retard their growth, they may even kill a few, but in the end it is the body itself that must destroy what organisms are left, must clean up the battlefield, seek out and destroy that last final microbe. No matter where the organism is hidden or lodged, in the end, now as always, it is the body that must do the final killing. All the great medical breakthroughs in infectious diseases, all the drugs and technical achievements have done nothing more than assist the body's own immune system. They give us an edge, the time to mount a defense; in reality they do nothing more.

We have all been lulled into a sense of security by medical achievements, as if the achievements themselves are the answer. But nothing works for the baby born with immunodeficiency disease. The drugs the pediatrician prescribes to clear this infant's mouth do not work. Despite all the efforts, despite the mycostatin, the gentian violet, all the drugs that are used, the swabbing of the gums, lips and inner cheeks, the fungus continues to grow. Horrified, the parents watch while medicine fails. They see the grayish plaques creep down the front of their baby's face, out of his nose. They watch it spill out onto his chin and neck. The plaques begin to crack and bleed, the round, pudgy face becomes distorted. Hungry, yet unable to eat, the baby struggles and squirms; his mouth begins to rot. The fungus starts down the back of his throat, down his esophagus into his stomach. He begins to cough up blood.

The physician may by now know what is wrong or he may have called the university. The doctors there can't be sure but they make a presumptive diagnosis of combined immunodeficiency, Swiss type, agammaglobulinemia. They caution the physician against giving a smallpox vaccination. It is also recommended that the patient be transferred to the university. The doctor tells the parents, but without being told, without even knowing what the word immunodeficiency means, they know. It is obvious to them, as it is to everybody else now, that their baby is in a desperate battle. His body, silently, frantically, is fighting for its life.

The child has been transformed and to these parents, bitter and confused, worn down by weeks of concern and fear, emotionally drained, it seems that nature gone blind now goes mad. They sit in the university conference room listening to the professor of immunology, their son's new doctor, tell them that their child cannot make the antibodies necessary to fight infections. He doesn't have the white cells necessary to destroy the foreign attackers entering his body; he has no lymphocytes to fight cellular invaders.

"But what does that mean?" the father asks.

"It means," the professor says, "that your baby cannot defend himself against microscopic invaders such as bacteria, viruses and fungi. I am a pediatric immunologist and that's why your child was referred by your doctor here to my department and not to the department of cardiology, neurology or renal disease."

"Can you do anything?" the mother asks. "I mean, with Freddie?"

The professor doesn't answer.

The father looks at him skeptically. "A little, but not enough. Right?"

Even while they are talking, the patient as a new admission is being examined by the chief resident. Scrawny, the child has not gained any weight in the last month. His mouth is so cracked and sore he cannot suck. His ears are filled with pus, his eyes inflamed. His chest film is positive for a right middle-lobe pneumonia; there are abscesses under his arms and in his groin. Even without eating, his bowels explode with greenish-white diarrhea, continually soiling the examining table.

"Some of the problems of working at a large medical referral center like this one," the professor explains, "are that for all our expertise, it is a hospital of last resort. By that I mean the patients who finally do get here have had, like your son, a confusing picture, and parents, like yourselves, by the time they sit down in this room have been through it all already. They have been told one story after another. Like you, they have gone through tests that didn't prove anything, had diagnoses given that weren't correct, medicines prescribed that didn't work. In many cases they, like yourselves, have been on their own, stopping drugs because the drugs they were told to use obviously didn't work, or just switching back to an old one because their baby took it better than the newer one. We've even had parents here whose doctors have refused to admit they didn't know what was wrong. Told the family there was nothing to worry about, or sent them to somebody else who did the same things that had been done before all over again, only adding more medications and perhaps some more tests. All getting the parents and their babies nowhere. Many parents have gone through two or three rounds of physicians before they get here.

"I'm not defending the deficiencies of medicine, but there are some diseases where the diagnosis is not as evident as we would like to think. Diseases that at the beginning can look like many other conditions. Since some may be quite benign, the only chance we have at diagnosis is simply waiting and watching. Things are pretty easy for both the doctor and the patient when it's a broken leg or appendicitis. The diagnosis is obvious; it's made and the condition is fixed. But your child's problem, the real reason that he's been so ill and for so long, was not that easy to find out. He has a rare condition, not as rare as we would like, but rare enough to make the right diagnosis difficult. We see perhaps five children a year here with a problem similar to your son's, and we draw our patients from an area of over seven states. Your average doctor in practice may not see a single child with such a condition during all of his professional life, not one.

"Yet none of the problems that your son has are medically unique in themselves. They all happen in some degree to every baby. Every infant has colds, ear infections. Every baby somewhere, sometime in his infancy has infectious diarrhea, and a lot have thrush. Every newborn and infant is susceptible to the organisms that cause these conditions.

"Nothing that has happened to your baby has not happened to others. His problem is not that he gets these things, but that once he gets them he cannot turn them off. He does not have the ability to destroy the organisms that affect him, so the infections smolder along or, like the fungus in his mouth, they just keep growing. He gets recurrent infections. His inability to handle bacteria, viruses and fungi has nothing to do with the type of infecting organism. He cannot handle any of them, no matter what they are.

"Your son was born with a congenital defect," the doctor continues. "Like a heart that did not form right. The organs necessary to protect him from microorganisms simply did not develop. It is not your fault, it is not something you did or didn't do. No drugs that you might have taken during your pregnancy caused this, or anything you did or ate or didn't do or didn't eat while you were carrying him. It is, though, a congenital defect, and like any other congenital defect it means that a part of your son's body which should have developed while he was being formed didn't. Just as children born with congenital heart defects have trouble running or may turn blue, children with congenital kidney defects may swell up, and those with congenital abnormalities of the nervous system can expect to have seizures and learning disabilities, your child born without an immune system ends up fighting one infection after another and losing.

"All the coughs he's had, all the colds, all the diarrheas, the crankiness, the ear infections, the fungal infection in his mouth,

[14]

the trouble breathing and feeding, his inability to gain weight, all of it is because he does not have the chemical system that our body needs to defend us against attacks by foreign organisms. That is his real disease, the real cause of his problems—no defense system. And it is really a system, a whole group of different organs working separately, yet developing together, doing different things but all with one goal—bodily defense against microbes. Just as the heart and great vessels are made up of different parts, and a defect in any one of these parts can lead to the different kinds of congenital heart defects, there can be different kinds of immune deficiencies too.

"Some children have different parts of the system absent. Some lose the parts that produce the circulating antibodies; others have the circulating antibodies but not all the types of white cells that are needed to eat up the different kinds of organisms. There are children who have normal circulating antibodies and one kind of normal white cells called granulocytes, but lack the other type of white cells we call lymphocytes. And each lack or deficiency presents itself clinically to the doctor and to the parents in its own particular way. No antibodies, and the child has recurrent pneumonias and abscesses; no granulocytes, and he has prolonged bacterial infections; no lymphocytes, and he has recurrent fungal infections and severe recurrent, almost unending viral illnesses, chickenpox and mumps that can be so severe as to be life-threatening. The antibody part of our immune system we call our humoral defense system; the white-cell part, our cellular defense. There are other helpers around, but these two really make up almost all of our immune system."

"And our son?" the father asks.

"We're fairly sure right now from his history and a few of the tests that have already been done by your family doctor that he has none of the parts, that he has no immunologic defenses at all."

"So he's the worst, then."

The doctor hesitates. "Yes, I'm sorry, I'm afraid your son is the worst."

"What can we expect?"

"There is not much we can do. Antibiotics really only work

against bacterial infections if the body's own defenses are in order. Against viruses we really can do nothing and never could. That is totally left up to the body itself."

"And so?"

"He will eventually acquire an infection—a meningitis, a pneumonia, a tonsillitis—that will be too much for him, and he will die from that overwhelming infection, whatever it is."

"How long?"

"No more than two years."

"And he'll be sick the whole time?"

"Yes."

"Never normal?"

"I'm afraid not."

There is not a sound in the room. The father, stroking his head, sits and stares at the floor.

"Is there nothing that can be done?" the mother asks.

"Well, there may be, but right now it is very experimental. In fact," the doctor says almost reluctantly, "it has never been used on humans."

The father looks up. "What is it?" he asks.

"It is what we call a bone-marrow transplant. The cells that manufacture antibodies and the cells that eventually become the various kinds of white cells all come from primitive cells that begin in the marrow of our bones. The idea of bone-marrow transplants is to take these cells from a normal person and transplant them into the bone marrow of an immunodeficient child, and hope they will grow more—in a sense, hope that they will replace his absent system."

"Well?" the father asks impatiently.

"It works at least in some animals, but in others, even though the transplanted cells do take, do grow in the recipient's own bone marrow, when they reach a certain density they begin to attack the tissues of their host.

"It is as if these donor cells were rejecting their host, rather than the usual other-way-around where the recipient rejects the transplant, and in this reverse process the recipient dies, is taken over and finally destroyed by the transplanted, immunologically competent bone marrow of the donor. It is called a graph-versus-host rejection. It would be very risky . . ."

"I don't care," the mother says. Filled with despair and

grief, with a sense of the uncertainty of human life, she asks what mothers have always asked, the question that has given medicine its strength and its burden, that is older than love itself.

"Doctor, can you save him?" she pleads. "Can you save my baby?"

2

In the Beginning

THE SCIENCE OF IMMUNOLOGY is barely a hundred years old, but the processes it deals with are as old as the earth itself. The way our bodies fight infections began even as the earth was cooling. It has evolved along with the oceans and the continents, so that today the antibodies that patrol our circulation, the white cells that guard our tissues are as fundamental as the rocks we walk on and the air we breathe.

The fluids in our bodies mimic the primeval seas in which we began. The concentrations of salts, of sodium, potassium and chloride in our bloodstream, the cobalt, magnesium and zinc in our tissues, are the same as those that existed in the earliest seas.

We still carry those seas within us, and the same chemical battles that were fought in them a billion years ago are being waged today in fighting our infections and controlling our illnesses. The battlefields may have shrunk from hundreds of square miles of ocean to a few cubic centimeters of blood, from bays and inlets to the fluids of kidneys and lungs, but failure then meant the same as it does now—decay and destruction, the end of all that had gone before and all that might have come after.

Not only does our blood go back to those ancient seas; we are also, literally, children of the earth. The carbon in our bones is the same carbon that forms the rocks of the oldest mountains. The molecules of sugar that flow through our bloodstream once flowed in the sap of now fossilized trees, while the nitrogen that binds together our bones is the same nitrogen that binds the nitrates to the soil. Life has endured as long as it has because it is formed from substances as basic as the earth itself.

Nobody knows when life first appeared. For that matter, nobody knows what life is. All we really know is that somewhere in the long continuous evolution of the oceans there came a moment so basically different from the moment before, from all the moments before, that in that instant, despite everything being physically the same—the same depth, the same volume, the same salinity, the same weight and concentration of salts, the same percentage of dissolvable materials, the same tides and drifts and currents—those seas were suddenly not the same at all.

There is an idea most of us share, that whatever it was which began in that distant time was a very fragile thing. It is a notion nourished by our humanity and our fears, but also it has been fostered by science itself. Unable not only to define what life is but to explore its parts without destroying what is being searched for, the scientist defends his failure by conjuring up the view that life is a delicate mechanism, that what he is dealing with is a tenuous structure so precariously balanced that even the tiniest insult can shatter it.

Yet whatever it was that happened in those ancient seas has endured. Ages have come and gone, land masses have shifted, the geography of the oceans has changed, oxygen has permeated the atmosphere, temperatures have risen and fallen and risen again, yet through it all, despite its seeming fragility, life has survived and prospered. It has filled the earth and the skies, it exists in the deepest parts of the oceans and clings to the highest mountains.

LIFE'S BEGINNINGS may be shrouded in mystery, the miracle that brought it about may be hidden forever. But perhaps the greatest mystery is not its beginnings but its incredible tenacity. Life's endurance, its survival, growth and domination—these are qualities as rare as its birth, and of these we do indeed know something.

[19]

Our earth, it is estimated, began some four billion years ago. If there was no passion in its making, then it came about in the grim fastness of heat and fire. What stupendous catastrophe produced its beginning, what other worlds had to be consumed, what galaxies wrecked so that here in our corner of the Milky Way a new world might be born, can only be imagined.

Whatever the cause, it is conjectured that at that approximate four-billion-year date the flaming mass which was eventually to become our earth was torn from the surface of the sun and hurled spinning into space with such gigantic force that it did not come to rest for almost a hundred million miles where, in the midst of galactic dust and debris, it began finally to cool and condense.

All that is here on earth today was there then. Every element from argon to mercury, all the magnesium, lead, zinc, and carbon, all the iron and cadmium, all the gold and silver that was eventually to be in the oceans and in the ground were already there, superheated and uncombined, in that original molten mass.

The processes that brought life about, and continue to maintain it, began as the globe, rotating slowly in the vastness of space, began to cool. The elements, no longer kept apart as they had been by the heat of the mother sun, began slowly to combine one with the other. As the temperature on the molten surface dropped, chemistry took over. The atoms of hydrogen and oxygen swirling in the heat came together to form water; great clouds of it, kept in the atmosphere as superheated steam, circled the cooling globe. Nitrogen and hydrogen combined to form ammonia gas, while burning methane bubbling up from the red-hot carbides added to a haze so poisonous that even without the extreme heat, life would have been impossible.

As the earth continued to cool, the heavier elements began settling out, floating on its fiery surface, while the lighter metals rose and fell as incandescent vapors in the drifts of steam. Violent electrical storms raged across the earth's surface, and through the cracks appearing in the ever hardening crust, tons of molten carbon and iron geysered up into the glowing atmosphere.

All this is not mere speculation; it is a physical certainty.

Just as we are able to tell the age of the earth by the rate of its atomic decay, we know now exactly what happened as it gradually cooled.

In the early nineteen-fifties, scientists at the University of California simulated the conditions of that immensely remote period. They filled a bell jar with an atmosphere of heated methane, carbon dioxide, water vapor and ammonia, and sent currents of electricity through these gases. Out of the mixture came hundreds upon hundreds of complicated organic compounds. From a bell jar containing three simple gases saturated with nothing more than superheated water vapor came sugars and alcohols, amino acids, aldehydes, ketones and organic acids —the building blocks of life.

In the poisonous air of that bell jar, compounds were produced that today are found only in living creatures. The importance of the experiment was not that complicated organic molecules could be produced from simple gases, but that those molecules could and did come from an atmosphere which was, gas for gas, the atmosphere of our earth as it cooled down through the temperatures of superheated steam. It proved that the organic compounds which today we associate only with life, which we used to say could only come from living organic processes, were produced long before there was any chance for life at all; life came from these compounds, not the other way around. It meant that for over a billion years the earth itself formed the hydrocarbons, the amino acids, the sugars and ketones that would eventually become life's clay, not in the ounces or grams that were produced in the bell jar of the experiment but in the staggering amounts of trillions and trillions of tons. Today's oil reserves, the billions of barrels locked into the earth's crust, represent only a small percentage of the total amount of carbon compounds that were formed during the time of heat, vapor, electrical storms and simple gases.

Eventually, the surface of the earth had cooled enough for the water, so long held in the atmosphere as steam, to condense. Great curtains of rain began to drench the still-smoldering earth, a continual torrent washing out the atmosphere, cleansing it of the trillions of tons of compounds that had been formed there, carrying the sugars and ketones, alcohols and aldehydes down into the newly developing oceans.

[21]

It is important to bear in mind that during those hundreds of millions of years when organic compounds were formed in the atmosphere and later were being washed down into the seas, the earth itself was sterile. There was no life, no bacteria, no viruses, no plants, no algae, just a heated atmosphere of rain and a cooling globe slowly filling with warm oceans. It was in those waters that the sugars, the fats, alcohols and amino acids which today would have been oxidized or eaten by organisms —destroyed as soon as they were formed—survived.

What came after was a time of struggle, of survival of the fittest. Not the survival of any living creatures—there were none yet—but of what those creatures would ultimately be formed from, the organic molecules themselves.

The thousands of organic compounds which had been washed out of the atmosphere gathered in the coastal inlets and shallow tidewater pools of the developing oceans. The sugars and alcohols, the aldehydes and amino acids, the fats and carbohydrates which were the least stable slowly began coming apart, their fragments mingling with other dissolved debris, while the most stable of each chemical class remained and by default triumphed. There must have been whole lines of compounds that for a time seemed dominant, only eventually to disappear. Thousands of different kinds of sugars, hundreds of different alcohols, scores of dissimilar aldehydes, all had been washed down into the oceans, forming in the tidewater areas what has been called the "primeval soup." The molecules which survived that soup, those sugars which triumphed over the other sugars, those classes of alcohols which outlived their brothers, the amino acids that did not degenerate, gradually accumulated.

The compounds which survived did so for a number of reasons. The stability of how they were made, the number of atoms in them, the types of bonds holding these atoms together, even the molecule's shape and configuration, bore on survival. At length those chemically best suited to the ocean's own developing chemistry, the compounds most stable in the seas' own concentrations of acids and salts, were the ones which won the battle.

The biochemical struggles that went on in those warm,

sterile waters were as ruthless, as deadly as any battle for survival since; only the strongest made it. The molecules which would give rise to life were not a haphazard array of compounds indiscriminately thrown together, but those which had the physical strength, the chemical tenacity and endurance to survive the grueling, prolonged period of chemical evolution. Before life began, those organic compounds that were weak or would have eventually weakened were destroyed. The life that developed from the survivors began on a foundation already stable and already enduring.

Scientists are essentially in agreement about the processes that led to the formation of the organic molecules from which life finally came. It is on the question of what happened after their formation, and the gradual thinning out of the unstable compounds, that scientific speculation and confusion begins. Which came first, the chicken or the egg? Crystallization or precipitation? Colloid growth or gel formations?

All we can really be sure of is that the chemical processes which go on in our own bodies, the compounds that make up our metabolic pathways, the sugars and fats that carry our energy, the amino acids that constitute our proteins, the phospholipids that make up our cell walls, are the best compounds that nature could develop. We have within us the victors in a billion years' battle for survival.

No one knows how it happened, or precisely when, but those chemicals which did survive the struggle for existence must ultimately have formed themselves together into polymers—large molecules made up of a series of identical subunits. There is a distinct evolutionary advantage to size and complexity in that it allows for reaching across an area to gather in new substances, and for being too big to be easily destroyed. As the raw organic materials in the early seas thinned out, the competition which had existed among the simpler molecules continued with the polymers. Again, whole species of these molecular chains must have come and gone until finally, under the pressure for greater size and stability, enzymes came into existence. Evolving from polymers, these long-chained compounds could replicate and form more of themselves from the raw materials around them, from the carbon fragments, phosphates, sodium and chloride drifting in the oceans, rather than having to rely for growth on the linking together of already formed and completed sub-units.

The evolutionary advantage of enzymes over polymers is obvious. But survival and dominance meant more than simply continuing to grow, or merely to exist; it meant protecting whatever growth had been won. Without protection, the original organic molecules would have continually replaced one another until the cooling earth and changing seas eventually destroyed them all, winners and losers alike. There would have been no evolution. At best, evolution would have been nothing more than an endlessly repeating cycle of one uncomplicated molecular species gradually replacing a less suitable one until the cooling earth or changing seas, gradually becoming more and more physically inhospitable, at some point simply ended the whole thing.

Systems need protection to develop. Indeed, in the chemical evolution that immediately preceded life, protection was the crucial factor. Without protection for all the marvelous machinery of life to be gradually assembled, all the metabolic pathways to develop and be finally coupled—so that in a sea of increasing change and scarcity, the by-products of one enzymatic process might be used to feed another—life could never have occurred. Without protection, no organic system could have been built. There would have been no time for refinements of organization, no slow process of trial and error, no interconnecting of different metabolic cycles, no use of one part by another, no evolutionary movement on which to build.

Protection preceded life. A molecule with a bit of clay on its surface was better sheltered from destructive cosmic rays than one without such protection. A polymer that had chemical groups on it to repel attacks of acid ions would continue to exist, even though the alkalinity of the sea changed. An enzyme with its active sites shielded from heat would continue to function long after its less fortunate neighbors. The means of protection varied, but they became as crucial an ingredient to survival as chemical efficiency itself. The same slow evolutionary tenacity that went into the making of a better polymer and a more structurally sound enzyme went into the development of defenses. What finally came out of those primeval waters may not have been solely the result of protective mechanisms, but it was surely sustained and maintained by them.

Life and protection have always gone hand in hand, and the two have been so closely intermingled that we sometimes fail to see the connection. The evolutionary formation of membranes was the first truly dramatic example of this intertwining. Membranes are by far the most efficient way of distributing large surface areas over short distances. In the chemical competition that preceded life, the formation of membranes from the already existing polymers and enzymes was a logical step to greater metabolic efficiency. But these membranes served another and perhaps more important purpose—protection.

Now there was finally a clear way to divide the outside from the inside. The ability to keep the outside out and the inside in gave a new and virtually indestructible stability to the molecules and enzymes that had been evolving in the open seas. The amino acids, alcohols, DNA, RNA, histones and sugars which because of their own strength had survived while other, less suited molecules had perished, now enclosed by these new membranes, were assured an environment in which they would always be dominant. The ancient seas, just as they were then, were suddenly and forever preserved. By the simple expedient of separating tiny parts of the oceans from the whole, of containing these parts within the membranes, they and their contents were once and for all kept apart from the changing salt concentrations, from the increasing minerals and alkalinities, and from the sludge draining off the continents. Those first seas were maintained, and the molecules within them granted an unchanging perpetual existence unaffected by external environmental forces.

Within those seemingly delicate membranes, many no more than one half of a micron thick, a whole world was sequestered away. No longer would time or temperature affect its waters. Ice ages would come and go, the oceans would fill with materials, lakes would form, the very air would change, and still the ancient seas would go on and on undisturbed, unchanging, allowing life to develop in an environment to which its parts were already eminently suited, and were totally secure.

Membranes, which seem to have won their place in chemical evolution because of their ability to bring many different chemical processes together in a very small area, really succeeded because of the protection they gave. It was not a new kind of chemical process or method, but a new kind of defense which, by securing within it all that chemical evolution which had already been won, allowed evolution to go on.

We tend to ignore the concept of protection, or think of it as secondary to the intricacies of life. Yet as much intricacy and sophistication has gone into the protection of life as into the development of photosynthesis, or the process that carries oxygen to our brains. Indeed, the highest development of the chemistry that began in the heat and the steam of the earth's primitive atmosphere may not be life itself, but the marvelous ability which has developed to protect it. This day and every day we each carry within us not only the most sophisticated of life processes but also the most stunningly effective protection the world has ever seen, the end result of an evolution as complicated and as intricate as life itself—our immune system.

WE LIVE TODAY as we always have, at the bottom of a sea of bacteria and viruses. They have evolved with us every step of the way. They swam beside us even before we could breathe. As cells, we fought them for bits of food, and then, a billion years later, for our very lives. No matter how we may wish to view ourselves, despite all our fantasies of grandeur and dominion, all our fragile human successes, the real struggle once chemical evolution ended has always been against bacteria and viruses, against adversaries never more than seven microns wide. In the battle for species survival it has been our immune system, more than all of our other strengths and assets, more than our hands, our speed and agility, even more than our minds, that has sustained us and allows us to endure for whatever ends.

Once the chemistry of life was firmly protected within cell membranes, the evolution we are familiar with—the evolving of living creatures—began, and with it the beginning of our immune system.

To be sure, chemical evolution itself went on during the evolution of living things. New and more efficient systems continued to develop, metabolic processes became more efficient. Cycles evolved within the membranes themselves, helping them to maintain their structural integrity against any sudden chemical changes in the surrounding seas. Plant photosynthesis began, bacterial metabolism turned from the anaerobic state to the more efficient and more powerful aerobic respiration, more stable proteins were synthesized, stronger walls and membranes were produced, and high-energy phosphates began flooding the developing cells, providing a new fuel able to drive the newer and more expansive cellular processes.

Life was already secure. It might easily have gone on as it had first evolved, surviving on its primitive machinery—single elementary cells, barely alive yet growing, slowly making more of their own kind. But by the time of cellular life, a new pressure had entered those early oceans—the need for food. In a sea of increasing scarcity, the cell which could better utilize energy sources to maintain itself would prosper, and in that prospering, force out the less efficient cells. So life, driven now by the need for food, continued to evolve. Any random change in any cell, any mutation that increased the ability of an enzyme to give its cell access to more energy, or a better transfer of energy, that allowed for a more efficient utilization of old food sources or the use of new ones, became established and endured.

Dead ends occurred. One is still with us today—primitive sulfur-using cells locked forever in the depths of the ocean, cells that had learned to metabolize sulfur for energy and had prospered for a while, only to be displaced by the more efficient photosynthetic cells that powered their own internal systems and reproduced more of themselves by using the sun itself as an energy source; sulfur was in limited supply, the sun was not. Photosynthetic cells eventually filled the world, while the sulfur cells stayed and still stay where they were.

By the time photosynthesis evolved, the earth had cooled to well below 100 degrees. All the organic compounds that had been formed earlier, when the earth was hotter, had long since been incorporated within membranes, into cellular machinery, or had been used up themselves as energy sources. The only truly available source of energy other than the sun was the organic substances being made within the cells themselves.

The seas, too, had become hostile. Minerals draining off the land masses had changed the concentrations of the salts to toxic levels. Amounts of dissolved oxygen had affected the acid-base balance, so that even those sugars and fats which might leak out of damaged or dying cells were themselves destroyed and unable to be used as food. The only food source large enough to fuel evolution was locked up within the cells themselves, and so evolution took a violent turn.

Feeding began, and with that feeding came murder. Violence was suddenly everywhere. Whole species of organisms devoured the species next to them, only to be eaten themselves in turn. In terrible exchanges, chemistry gave way to defense, defense to chemistry, chemistry back again to defense; death became as important as life.

The organisms that eventually survived triumphed not only because of differences in their metabolism, a greater ability to utilize available foods, but because of their aggressiveness and bodily defenses. Those that moved more quickly survived the slower; those that were too sticky to be torn apart continued to exist; those that fought back, that made poisons and chemicals which killed the organisms that were trying to kill them, went on to form more of their own. The battles were no longer for dominance but for sheer existence. And those struggles which began back in those early seas, when the first cell turned on its brother, have never ceased.

3

Forerunners: The First Insights

THE CONCEPT OF MEDICINE is as old as man's suffering. Yet whatever paths medicine may have taken in its long history, however much some men might have tried to profit from it, to divert it from its true course—it has always managed to retain its worth, to sustain its value by going back time and again to its roots, to the plea for help that first called it into being, to that first "Doctor, can you save my baby?"

As with any sustained human effort, medicine has seen a constant revision of "knowledge" by facts, the new replacing the old, and the old forever going down hard. The battles of medicine have been epic, at times vicious affairs, but the most brutal, those that have ruined men and wrecked careers, have not been fought by doctors against charlatans or myths or superstitions, or against laymen who for whatever reasons wished to stop progress; they have been fought by physicians against physicians. What is at issue in these battles is always the same: doctors forgetting or ignoring their oath, substituting dogma for experience, theory for the bedside. Eventually they are challenged by others who are unable to ignore the suffering and the grief they see about them, who never cease to respond to the pleas for help and stubbornly hold to their vision of something better, of a more effective, more reasonable type of medicine.

Some, like Semmelweis, do so at the expense of their lives; he refused to yield to the pressure of his colleagues and was driven insane. Harvey, from the moment of the publication in 1628 of his monumental *Essay on the Motion of the Heart and the Blood,* was opposed. Many of his patients deserted him, while professional colleagues attacked his theory. As late as forty years after his publication on the circulation of the blood, his ideas, challenged by the professors teaching Galenic medicine, were still refused general acceptance. Two hundred years later, Jenner's belief that vaccination could protect people from the ravages of smallpox was initially attacked, so that he felt compelled at great personal expense to publish his own monograph to communicate his findings and interpretations. Koch, working without academic support, developed by himself the techniques of modern microbiology. Pasteur, one of the greatest scientists of all time, ran the risk of indictment for murder in his use of the rabies vaccine. Yet he persisted, defying accepted beliefs and practices to save a life.

Progress in medicine has always been rooted in impulses and insights unrelated to anything but a passion for the truth, although the truth may at first be only vaguely sensed, and may for the most part be the consequence of facts and reasons that are not clear to the discoverer himself. These medical insights and impulses are extraordinary events that in the end affect every one of us. Nowhere can such insights and the struggles of medicine be more clearly seen than in the development of immunology.

That study had its beginnings in the discipline of infectious diseases. It was a few early medieval physicians, concerned with the spread of plagues, who might be called pioneers in the field. Trying to understand why some were spared the pain and suffering of contagion while others died feverish and consumed within days, they made the initial observations and contributions which in the present century culminated in the new science of immunology, the greatest healing science ever developed.

The idea that disease is caused by living things reproducing themselves, yet too small to be seen, is not a modern concept. It began centuries ago, at a time when diseases were considered due to a malfunction of the four "humors" of the body—blood, phlegm, yellow bile and black bile—and when the five "entia" were assumed to affect all human life—the stars, food, the mind, divine purpose, and poisons. It was the time when boiling oil was poured into gunshot wounds to protect against the evil humors of gunpowder, turning the wounded into life-long cripples and courageous troopers into raving lunatics, even though the doctors themselves pouring the pitch observed "those burnt with the scaly oil were made terrible swolne." Physicians in the lecture halls of the greatest medical schools of Europe spent their time and energies discussing which of the precious stones —sapphires, emeralds or pearls—when put into wine had the greatest therapeutic value.

But one man, fighting all the superstitions and traditions of his day, had the courage to declare in 1546 that "infection itself is composed of minute and sensible particles and proceeds from them." Geographer, astronomer, poet, musician, mathematician, biologist and physician, Fracastorius watched typhus, bubonic plague, syphilis and smallpox ravage his age. He was an acute observer who saw the need for releasing medicine from the shackles of dogma, and returning it to the realms of reason and experience. He became a clinician in the true sense of the word, and distinguished for the first time the three basic forms of contagium: diseases like leprosy spread by simple contact, epidemics like bubonic plague spread indirectly through contact with inanimate objects such as clothing and bedsheets, and plagues like smallpox transmitted over long distances without any apparent personal or inanimate contact direct or indirect between those afflicted.

In a world of Aristotelian formalism and religious dogma, where physicians blindly followed the centuries-old rules of Galen, Fracastorius looked with open eyes. "There are diseases of plants which do not contaminate animals," he wrote, "and vice versa animal diseases which do not attack plants. There are other diseases restricted to man or to certain animals such as cattle and so on; certain diseases have affinity for certain individuals as they do for certain organs. If we consider these contagiums intuitively we shall see that the contagium of a putrefaction goes from one body to another whether adjacent or distant. These seeds have the faculty of multiplying and propagating rapidly." But in the end the pressures of tradition, self-service and arrogance defeated Fracastorius, and the world went back to witch-hazel nuts for fever, to smelling urine for diagnosis, and to bloodletting for pneumonias.

The battles have always been the same. "Very few physicians," wrote Paracelsus, a sixteenth-century physician and scholar making the same fight as Fracastorius, "have exact knowledge of diseases and their causes, but my books are not written like those of other physicians, merely copying the ancient authorities. I have composed them on the basis of experience, which is the greatest master of everything, and with indefatigable labor. Look," he pleaded with physicians, "observe, go back to the bedside; be suspicious of eloquence, ignore ceremony, lecture and write in the common language, proceed from reason and move on the learning of experience." And for those words the greatest physician of his century was excluded from university halls, ridiculed by professors, persecuted by his enemies, unable to find a printer to publish his writings or a university to acknowledge his findings. Like all the great medical innovators, Paracelsus was the butt of the most infamous accusations. With patients dying about him, pain going on unrelieved, suffering and grief a way of life, he was regarded as a heretic worthy of dying at the stake. Like any man of great integrity willing to make a stand because he feels he is right, he was attacked and hounded. He survived but his ideas died, buried along with those of Fracastorius.

Three hundred years later, in what might be thought the more enlightened nineteenth century, when Aristotle and Galen were no longer used as authorities but other theories, other doctrines of the day, were as blindly and rigidly followed, another courageous physician was attacked with the same self-serving ridicule, the same pompous abuse, the same professional hounding.

This time it was not an established physician but a young doctor, an assistant professor in the First Obstetrical Clinic in the Lying-In Hospital in Vienna, named Semmelweis. Later to be considered one of the greatest benefactors of humanity, he was destroyed as much by his grief at going unheeded as by the abuse of his colleagues, while for the want of simple hand washing with an antiseptic solution of chlorinated lime he advised, women were buried after their deliveries instead of being blessed. This time the idea survived the man, and anyone who has taken his wife home from a maternity ward safe and alive is reaping the benefits of Semmelweis' beliefs.

Medicine had progressed in the four centuries from Paracelsus to Semmelweis, but the progress had been slow and inconstant. Fabricated treatments, medical superstitions, false texts, outdated methods of teaching vied constantly with truth, reason and concern. The Greek concept of blood moving between the chambers of the heart through invisible pores was accepted by the medical community well after the studies of Da Vinci, Vesalius and Harvey proved it false. That the body was but the instrument of the soul was accepted long after Galileo showed the effectiveness of the experimental method. Applications of heat to cure diseases that came from cold, and cold compresses for diseases that came from heat, pepper for fever, parsley and celery for chills, bleeding considered revulsive when performed on a part of the body distant from the diseased part and yet derivative when done near the diseased organ—all this was still accepted dogma and standard treatment at the same time that Copernicus was proving the superiority of exact mathematical calculations over speculation, and Descartes a century later the weakness of the senses when compared to reason.

Medicine, jealous of innovation, continually abused its own; physicians were ostracized, ridiculed and even killed because they tried to free themselves from dogma and metaphysics, because they advocated the experimental method, proposed the observation of nature rather than reliance on ancient texts, because they attacked accepted doctrines or tried nothing more than a better way to relieve their patients' suffering. It has not ended. In every generation, including our own, there have been physicians who could well understand Harvey's anger and disgust when forty-three years after the publication of his description of the movement of the blood, still being attacked by other physicians for his views, he was forced to write:

"To return evil speaking with evil speaking, I hold to be

unworthy a philosopher and searcher after truth. I believe that I shall do better and more advisedly if I meet so many indications of ill-breeding with the light of faithful and conclusive observation. It cannot be helped that dogs bark and vomit their foul stomachs or the cynic should be numbered among philosophers, but care can be taken that they do not bite or inoculate their mad humors or with their dog's teeth gnaw the bones and foundations of truth. . . . Let them go on railing I say until they are weary if not ashamed."

Late-Renaissance physicians finally abandoned medieval doctrines; they became scientific observers. Medicine progressed, if progress can be measured by the raw accumulation of knowledge, the simple ledgering of isolated facts and observations. In 1665 Hooke, using razor slices of cork and the newly developed microscope, gave a brief description of the cellular nature of tissues, using the word "cell" for the first time. Leeuwenhoek described the presence in the blood of cellular elements that he called red cells. Porter, through the use of the opera glass, became convinced that vision was not due to rays leaving the eye but to something entering it. In 1761 Auenbrugger began listening to the chest; others followed and the various sounds of pneumonia, emphysema and tumors came to be distinguished. In the nineteenth century, blood pressure commenced to be taken, rheumatic fever was finally connected to heart disease, bile was recognized as important in the digestion of foods.

Yet if physicians were becoming scientists, medicine was not becoming a science. The body was still left to fend for itself; the fact that life and death, curing and healing, ultimately depended on the body and its own chemistry, its own defense, was not generally recognized. The chest may have been listened to and blood pressure taken, but the implications were not understood. Without knowledge of the cause of disease, without an understanding of pathology, treatment was merely faddism.

Reputations were made on specious reasoning and half-truths, and science became the new tyranny. Adopting what was considered to be the scientific method, physicians constructed faulty systems in an effort to explain disease on the basis of whatever was the newest discovery. Borelli, a pupil of Galileo's, taught that the human organism was merely a machine, that the soul was the effective cause of animal movements and that the soul brings about those movements through tugging on the muscles. Broussais, influenced by a few studies of gastroenteritis, based his whole theory of disease on nothing more than gastric distress; he advised the application of leeches to the stomach as treatment for all illnesses, and became respected for his theory and even wealthy. Mesmer, using the new concepts of magnetism, developed a whole theory of disease based solely on "animal magnetism," and had thousands of disciples. Purgatives were used by some to treat all illnesses. Opium was used so indiscriminately that it killed as many as it relieved; ipecac was prescribed for any kind of vomiting or diarrhea. Cinchona bark, useful only for malarial fever, was generally indicated for any kind of febrile illness.

The trend to experimentation, much as the same trend today, took the physicians away from the bedside, away from their patients, away from looking and seeing what indeed they were doing. Sydenham in the seventeenth century would have agreed with Bernard in the nineteenth: "One must break the bonds of philosophies and scientific systems as one would break the chains of scientific slavery. Systems tend to enslave the human spirit. Return to common sense, to practical methods."

Looked at coldly from what we know today, it made little difference whether the treatment for infectious diseases such as meningitis was purgatives or leeches. As recently as the early nineteen-forties, family physicians all over the world still waited patiently at the bedside, as they had always waited, for the fever of the pneumonia to break, having by then the sense to know that no matter what they did, if the fever broke, the patient would soon recover; if it did not, empyema, sepsis and death were a real possibility. They sat, too, by other bedsides, knowing, as physicians before them had always known, that no matter what was administered, the child with rheumatic heart disease would not live past the age of nine, that a 30 percent third-degree-burn victim was doomed, no matter what.

In other areas of medicine, ignorance was not so benign and occasionally it became murderous. The simple idea of cleanliness was one of these areas. Since there was always "good pus" coming from wounds as well as "bad pus," the proposal to use only clean bandages was scoffed at and ridiculed. Paré, in the sixteenth century, recommended that wounds be kept clean, washed with pure water and left to the open air. So did Paracelsus. But pus and decay had always been as much a part of early medicine and surgery as machines are today. They were the badges of the profession. Medical students walked around then as proudly in their blood-and-pus-stained aprons as today they hold up X-rays or flip around their new stethoscopes. For four hundred years physicians smelled, measured and weighed the pus to make their diagnosis. The struggle simply to get physicians to wash their hands and their instruments is one of the saddest episodes in the annals of medicine.

As LATE AS 1880 William Stewart Halsted, later to become the first professor of surgery at the new Johns Hopkins Hospital but then a young surgeon in residence at Bellevue, became incensed at his professor for refusing to wash his hands before an operation. Surgery was performed in an open wooden amphitheater, with the surgeons dressed in their street clothes. It was there in the pit of the amphitheater that Halsted, in his shirt sleeves, challenged Professor Jackson, impeccably dressed in his frock coat, to first wash his hands in a bowl of dilute carbolic acid before he began the surgery.

Halsted, independently wealthy, had just returned from a year of travel in Europe, and his visits to the great medical centers of Germany, France and Austria had convinced him that washing with dilute carbolic acid was the key to decreasing the appalling incidence of surgical wound infections. By the eighteen-eighties as many as 35 to 60 percent of all surgical cases were becoming infected. Surgical wards were literally turning into morgues. There were no antibiotics then, and the mortality from elective surgical postoperative wound infections —people dying from infections following the simplest operation, removal of a benign lymph node or a simple cyst—was staggering.

Thirty-five years before Halsted felt compelled, despite his junior status, to challenge his professor and risk dismissal from Bellevue, anesthesia had been discovered. With the horrible pain of surgery at last banished, surgeons were finally able to perform procedures that patients could not have tolerated before, and the surgeons pushed for all the traffic would bear.

Elective surgery was performed whenever possible—in a great number of cases when it wasn't even appropriate. Cysts were removed, growths excised, thyroids sectioned, benign skin tumors resected. In those thirty-five years, between the discovery of anesthesia and Halsted's travels, the number of operative procedures performed in surgical centers mounted to what were then incredible proportions, and with the increased number of operations came more deaths. People admitted to surgical wards for the removal of a simple, uncomplicated growth, perhaps not even enough to disfigure them, died two weeks later from a surgical wound infection. It was an unfortunate example of how a major medical achievement can lead directly to a major medical disaster.

Those surgeons who complained about the situation, who demanded better surgical selection processes or simply the taking of more care, were shouted down or ignored by their enthusiastic associates, who could now operate where and when they wished. The time of asepsis had not yet arrived, and at Bellevue in New York, surgical patients died in the corridors. From 1867 on, Lister in Scotland had published papers and given lectures showing that just washing hands and instruments could significantly lower the terrifying incidence of postoperative wound infections. But most surgeons, even faced daily with large numbers of their own patients becoming infected, and having to watch many of them die, still refused to believe. They agreed with Jackson, who angrily poured the carbolic acid out of the basin that Halsted had placed at the head of the operating table, ordered the "impudent" young surgeon out of "his" operating suite and began the operation, cutting into the breast of his young woman patient with his filthy hands and even filthier instruments.

Halsted survived and is remembered today as the first great surgeon in America; Jackson is remembered only for his arrogance. And the man who gave Halsted the facts he needed to challenge Jackson and eventually change American surgery was a Hungarian obstetrician in Vienna, Ignaz Philipp Semmelweis, who won with his own death Halsted's ultimate victory, and with Halsted's victory, our own.

In 1773 Charles White in his paper on the management of pregnant and lying-in women had written, as Hippocrates, Paré and Paracelsus had written before him, about the importance of cleanliness in childbirth. Indeed, he insisted upon the necessity of surgical cleanliness in his own hospital at Manchester, England. It was a time of hospital medicine. All over Europe great hospitals had been built; the drift of medicine had carried care out of the homes into these centers. It was here now that physicians were trained and treatments administered. Women for the first time began to be admitted to hospitals to deliver their babies. Lying-in hospitals were established, and with their establishment young mothers began to die in great numbers. Within days of their delivery a staggering proportion of these new mothers were suddenly dead.

Puerperal fever, as it was called (from the Latin *puer*, for child, and *parere*, to bear), is an infection of the uterus. The infecting organism, the streptococcus, is a bacterium which has evolved in its battle with our immune system a number of poisons that make it a difficult microbe for our bodies to destroy. It infects the womb of the postpartum woman, spreading rapidly along the womb's still-bleeding postdelivery surface, infects the fallopian tubes and then gets into the bloodstream, where it spreads rampantly throughout the whole body. There are fever, chills, seizures and heart failure, bleeding into the brain and kidneys, and then death within days, if not hours. So virulent was this type of streptococcal infection, so rapid its growth in the boggy, warm uterus that with barely the first signs of fever, over 50 percent of the women would be dead. In Lombardy alone it was reported that for a full year no woman survived childbirth. So great was the carnage that women pleaded not to be brought to the lying-in hospitals, to be allowed to deliver their babies at home. But the doctors insisted, the husbands agreed and the women died. It is hard now even to imagine why the obstetricians of those lying-in hospitals, seeing these women come into the hospital healthy and sound and then seeing them within days being taken to the morgue, did not at least stop the admissions.

Toward the end of the eighteenth century the infectious nature of puerperal fever was generally recognized. It would have taken a fool not to observe that these women were fine until delivery, that the deaths from the fever occurred only on the delivery wards, that the women in these obstetrical wards were dying in rows one after the other, all with the exact same symptoms, while women on other wards, not there to deliver babies, did not die. All kinds of theories were offered. Diet, for instance, was blamed as a cause of the fever, despite the fact that all the hospitalized patients, those who lived and those who died, ate the same food. Then the water was proposed, although there was no difference between the water drunk in the homes of the city where the delivering women didn't die and that drunk in the hospitals where they did. Some doctors even lectured to their students that it was the odor of certain flowers which caused puerpural fever; after all, there were more flowers on the maternity ward than on the other wards.

So the doctors did look for causes. They looked but they didn't see—all but one man. Self-service, the prestige of hospital medicine, the financial need to keep the obstetrical wards full, the personal convenience to the physicians of having all their patients delivered in one place, respect for the doctor, uncompromised belief in medicine—all won out. Doctors continued to admit women to the obstetrical wards, and thousands of women continued to consent or were made to.

Yet medicine had progressed. Autopsies were finally being done routinely. Virchow had pointed out the cellular basis of disease, and his histology, the study of diseased organs and tissues, had become a part of medicine by the time the problem of puerperal fever had begun.

Semmelweis discovered the cause of puerperal fever while routinely studying the post-mortem examination report of a pathology assistant, a colleague who had died of a hand wound obtained doing a dissection of a mother who had recently died of puerperal fever. During the autopsy, while dissecting out the diseased organ, the assistant had accidentally had his hand cut and within five days he, too, was dead. God knows what reasoning Semmelweis went through, why other physicians who read the same report and who like Semmelweis had seen other autopsies, did not come to the same conclusion he did.

History is full of intuitive guesses: Kekule understanding that carbon molecules could form rings, his insight opening up all of modern-day organic chemistry; Fleming looking at the bacterial culture plate and seeing the area surrounding the penicillin mold free of bacteria suddenly realizing that something from the mold had killed the bacteria; Madame Curie and uranium; Einstein sure without even knowing that time was not constant. It is such thoughts, against all accepted logic and reason, that are the true miracles of science. One of those understandings occurred to Semmelweis in his kerosene-lit study as he read that report. It suddenly came to him that the lesions in the organs of the dead pathology assistant—the bleeding vessels, the generalized hemorrhage, the abscesses and pus in the young man's body—were the same lesions that occurred in the bodies of the women dying from puerperal fever. But Kolletschka, the assistant, had not borne any child. The only injury he had incurred was a simple cut on his hand.

Semmelweis left his study and for the next few days traveled about Vienna, visiting other hospitals. He checked the death rates in the various obstetrical wards and found what he had feared and yet hoped. The death rates were highest in those hospitals where the physicians and medical students came on to the obstetrical wards directly from lectures on pathology or from dissecting rooms where they had handled the diseased organs of recently dead women. Kolletachka had cut his hand after handling such organs and he had died. Something on the hands—that was it! Those same hands, Semmelweis realized, hundreds a day, coming directly from the autopsy rooms, were being shoved by the physicians into the bleeding vaginas and torn wombs of delivering women. The hands—it was the hands! He could stop the plague.

Semmelweis went back to his own hospital, and demanded that the doctors coming from the autopsy rooms wash their hands before they did pelvic examinations or delivered any children. He was almost immediately attacked. Professors of obstetrics all over Europe, teachers in medical schools ridiculed him in the most brazen and brutal terms. The idea that disease could be introduced by the hands of a caring, competent physician was unthinkable, ridiculous. They refused to listen to him, called him crazy and deluded.

Even when he showed that in those few hospitals that still had two obstetrical services, one run by midwives and the other by physicians, the death rate from puerperal fever was practically zero on the wards where the midwives delivered the newborns and staggering on the wards where physicians did the deliveries—though the entrances to these wards were no more than a few feet apart—he was still attacked.

The doctors in his own hospital refused to wash their hands, but he persisted. There was no choice; driven by the daily horrifying spectacle of women dying unnecessary deaths, he cajoled, he pleaded with his colleagues. At first he was stunned by the obstinacy of his fellow physicians, who professed concern for their patients, yet continued on as they had, then he grew furious, and finally reckless. As death continued to follow death, as women, in the midst of what should have been joyfulness, warmth and love, vomited blood and died, raving, in their husbands' arms, he finally took to stationing himself in the doorway of his wards, physically forcing any physician who wanted to enter to wash his hands in a basin of dilute carbolic acid. There were fights and discussions of dismissal, but within months, while puerperal fever raged on in hospitals around them, there was not a single case of it on his wards. For the first time in fifteen years, the epidemic had been halted.

Semmelweis wrote up his findings, presented the data and was jeered. "How do you know it was the hand-washing?" the doctors said. "Maybe it was something else."

We all have our end points, those lines beyond which we cannot or will not pass. With the dismissal of his data, the refusal on the part of his contemporaries not only to believe but even to try his idea for a week or a day, an hour or even a minute, he went quietly, morbidly, insane. Still, the burden was too much for him; restrained, but hearing those screams in his head, the pleading of the young mothers to go home, to be allowed to deliver their babies somewhere else, not to be left to die, he struggled to free himself until his wrists and ankles, finally rubbed raw, became infected and he died.

That kind of anguish, the grief at being ignored and having others pay the price for your not being heard, the heartache of knowing you have something better to offer but that no one will even listen, has driven more physicians than Semmelweis insane—and not only in the distant past.

Barely twenty years ago Louis Pillemer, a young researcher at Yale, hounded by his contemporaries, went back to his lab and alone at night drank some of his Pento Barbitol Buffer and killed himself. He had made what would prove to be one of the major immunologic discoveries of this age, the beginning basis for a new understanding of how our bodies win the battle against microbial infections. But his findings of a strange protein in the blood that was not an antibody—indeed, as he proved, had nothing to do with antibodies but could nevertheless attack and destroy microorganisms—went against the accepted scientific antibody doctrine of the day. A nonimmunologic protein involved in what was obviously an immunologic function was unheard of. It challenged all the immunologic work being done at the time, undermined it, and the professors who had won their position by proposing the antibody theory would have none of it. Ridiculed and scoffed at, the researcher was attacked at scientific meetings, his papers were refused publication and his ideas were ignored. Today he is barely mentioned. When the protein he discovered—properdin—is discussed or taught, there may be an occasional vague reference to his name, but no more.

In the early eighteen hundreds Francisco Anterioacerbi, a pathologist, repeated in modern terms the words Fracastorius had written over three hundred years earlier: "The cause of contagious disease is specific organized substances capable of maintaining their own existence and of reproduction according to the common laws of all living things." Using the modern term "organized substance" rather than the sixteenth-century word "seeds" made no difference; like Fracastorius and the young Yale researcher, he was ignored.

IT IS CHASTENING and perhaps even humbling to realize that the very first demonstration, the first conclusive, unremitting proof that infectious diseases were not caused by vapors, curses or sin, that purgatives, leeches, mineral water, dry air or steam were not the least bit curative or for the most part even helpful in fighting infection, occurred no more than a little over one hundred and twenty-five years ago. The biologist, Agostino Bassi, having studied muscardine, a disease of silkworms, for over twenty-eight years, established that the disease was caused by "a living vegetative, cryptogamous parasite." He realized the implications of his discovery. Surrounded by dozens of foolish ideas about disease—none with a shred of logical or scientific support—he had shown beyond any doubt that one disease, muscardine, was caused by a live, infecting microorganism. In the silence of his laboratory, working at night at his bench dissecting the diseased silkworms and seeing the parasites infecting them, the whole of medicine, past, present and future, gradually became clear to him. The plagues, the wound infections, the horror of leprosy, the armies destroyed by typhus, the convulsions of rabies, the rotting brains of meningitis, pus-infected kidneys, destroyed hearts, women dying of puerpural fever—it was all one living thing eating another, even as it had been in the ancient seas.

Bassi took the intuitive lead, asserting—despite the opinion of his fellow physicians that he was making too much of one little silkworm, was "overstepping himself"—that many diseases of plants, animals and man are caused by animal and vegetable parasites. In 1864, still attacked, laughed at and abused, he wrote in much the same anger and exasperation as Harvey had written two hundred years before: "While many if not almost all eminent scientists believed and still believe that contagious materials are of a specific kind, they are actually living substances, that is to say animal, vegetable parasites." He refused to yield; others working in their own laboratories took up his cry; the greatest battle of medicine was finally being joined. Those who had ridiculed Semmelweis, who scoffed at the idea that disease could be spread by doctors themselves, were about to be defeated. But they went down hard.

From the eighteen hundreds on, science had been gathering momentum; the experimental method, rigorous controlled techniques, uncompromising skepticism pushed with ever increasing force against old dogmas and false new beliefs. After centuries of vacillation between alchemy and philosophy, mysticism and dogmatism, religion and rationalism, attempts to decide between hydrotherapy, diuretics, bloodletting, purgatives, no treatment or all treatments, medicine began gradually—first in bits and pieces and then finally in total—to rely on facts proved only by experience. Where once the academies with their metaphysical discussion had been the center of medical thought, then the clinics with their emphasis on diagnosis, then the hospitals with their concern for treatments, it now became the laboratory. It was there more and more that the attempts to solve disease and deal with illness were lodged.

[43]

The English physician John Snow was the first to prove, after centuries of human misery, that cholera was transmitted by polluted water, and thereby halted the London epidemic caused by water from the Broad Street pump in London in 1854. Working on his own, he encountered the almost total opposition of the medical establishment, even to the point of having to watch helplessly while one of his detractors drank the filthy water from the Thames to prove that good English water could not carry disease.

Bichat, in the course of doing over six hundred autopsies, had devised a whole new system of normal and abnormal pathology based on tissue rather than the archaic organ system that had been flourishing since the Middle Ages. The astonishing thing is that neither Snow nor Bichat used the microscope in their work, though the instrument had been available for over a hundred and fifty years.

In 1675 Leeuwenhoek had used the microscope to describe minute organisms, "little beasties," unseeable by the normal eye. Hooke had used it years later to describe the cell-like structures in his razor cuts of cork. The first satisfactory compound microscope, similar to the ones used today, was ready for use in the eighteen-twenties, yet it took another forty years for men with vision and audacity to take up Bichat's and Snow's concepts, and using the instrument definitively challenge the beliefs and concepts that had existed for over two thousand years. So profound were the microscopists' discoveries, so overwhelming the implications of what they found, so stunning and positive the applications of their knowledge that only today is medicine beginning to recover from their influence.

Koch, a general practitioner, using his office as a laboratory and a microscope to look at disease, began work that was to form the beginnings of the whole new science of bacteriology. Anthrax, a disease of hoofed animals, was epidemic in the region where he practiced. The infectious nature of the disease was obvious; whole herds went down in one area while in other provinces similar herds were spared. Koch, for the first time in history, worked out the life cycle of an infecting microbe, the anthrax parasite—a rod-shaped bacillus—proving that at one point in its life cycle it became a spore, a lifeless seed that covered the grasslands on which the animals fed. These seeds, he proved, would on ingestion by the animal turn again into the infecting bacillus, begin to multiply, eventually spreading throughout the animal's body, growing in every one of its organs, killing it. Koch published his report, and it was opposed. But support grew. His work was so self-evident, his technique so flawless and reproducible that after one short stupid academic battle his view won out.

Using the microscope and Koch's own methods for culturing bacteria, of obtaining pure cultures of bacterial growth, one disease-causing bacterium after another was discovered. Soon after the anthrax bacillus, the cholera bacillus was identified, then the diphtheria organism was isolated; the syphilitic spirochete, the tularemia microbe, typhoid, typhus, tetanus, tuberculosis all followed in short order. The new science of bacteriology was so dramatic in its findings, so impressively accurate in its discoveries, so definitive that for a time it threatened to take over all of medical science. Men with other thoughts and other concerns, other understandings and insights were silenced. Any study of pathology not having to do with the study of bacterial infections fell into disrepute; clinical observation and patient care gave way almost entirely to news from the laboratory. A new dogma, a new tyranny, began to develop and then finally to reign. Indeed, up to the present time, new voices have been silenced by it, new thoughts and ideas on disease dismissed or ridiculed.

Yet even at the beginning of this new revolution in medicine the seeds of doubt were present, a sense that not all diseases could be explained away by microbes. The achievements of the microbiologists and their successors, the infectious-disease experts, were stunning, the benefits to humanity almost miraculous, but it was not enough and some men knew it. Despite the new scientific paraphernalia of the medical laboratory —the culture mediums, the filters, the microscopes, the oil immersion lenses, the blood cultures—the bacteriologists could not for all their efforts find, for example, the organisms that cause rheumatic fever.

Rheumatic hearts were sectioned and studied for the microbes that supposedly caused the disease, but none were found. Tissues were examined microscopically, and re-examined, but even with the ever newer microscopic techniques and microbial stains, no bacteria were discovered. Blood from rheumatic children was injected into mice and guinea pigs, but the animals survived.

There was no apparent infecting organism in the children's bodies, yet they were ill. It was the same for cancer and the degenerative bone diseases, kidney disease, too—all left the infectious-disease experts baffled, as did the anemias. Still, dazzled by their own achievements, assured by their past successes, the new experts insisted that all diseases were caused by microbes, even those in which none could be found. They would be found, they insisted, eventually, if you just looked hard enough, developed better techniques or used more sophisticated devices.

The forest was again being lost for the trees. But there were men who probably never thought of themselves as being particularly courageous, men who, hearing the continuing cries for help, were again willing to brave the current tyranny and go beyond it.

4

Jenner and Pasteur

IT HAD BEEN KNOWN from antiquity that there were some diseases which, after they had once infected a person, never afflicted that person again, that injections of small amounts of certain poisons could render a person immune from larger unexpected doses. But it was Jenner, a modest medical practitioner of modest talent who literally single-handedly cleared our earth of one of the terrible scourges of mankind.

Jenner, working in the rural farmlands of England, became aware that women milking cows, milkmaids who had acquired cowpox, a mild smallpox-like disease contracted from cows, were spared the disfigurement of smallpox. That realization, one of the most momentous insights of medicine, is described in a contemporary biography in the most simple terms: "This event was brought about in the following manner. Jenner was pursuing his professional education in the house of his master at Sodbury. A young countrywoman came to seek advice. The subject of smallpox was mentioned in her presence. She immediately observed 'I cannot take that disease for I have had cowpox.' This incident riveted the attention of Jenner. It was the first time that the popular notion, which was not at all uncommon in the district, had been brought home to him with force and influence. Most happily, the impression which was then made was never effaced. Young as he was and insufficiently acquainted with any of the laws of physiology or pathology, he delved with deep interest on the communication which had been casually made known to him by a peasant."

Jenner undertook his experiment. He gathered the pus from the sore of a woman with cowpox and scratched it onto the arm of a healthy child. He watched the single simple pustule, the pox, develop and then, as expected with this mild disease, scab over and fall off. With what must have been great concern and perhaps even greater worry, he took the pus from an adult with smallpox and injected it into the child's skin. The child did not contract smallpox.

Jenner published his findings. But it was only one child, the critics said, and the publication of his work was attacked. He continued successfully to vaccinate more and more people, but still his views on the relationship between cowpox and the ability to resist smallpox continued to be challenged. After all, if vaccination with cowpox was so effective, how did it work? Jenner couldn't answer, but refusing to be silenced, he went on to make additional clinical observations ("Those who suffer from cold sores will not take the vaccination; it is best with them to wait until the cold sores are gone") on how to use what he knew was a valid treatment, indeed a miracle.

While the academic medical profession continued to insist that Jenner's insight was derived from an overinterpretation of wholly inadequate data, practitioners, seeing the terrible ravages of smallpox, listened to him and took up the procedure regardless of academic disapproval. The idea of vaccination spread and finally became established.

Jenner was the first man to use a live virus, related to though different from the human disease-causing virus, to protect mankind from illness. Today the Sabin polio immunization, the measles, mumps and German-measles vaccines are a continued reflection of Jenner's enormous contribution and courage to continue his work and to spread it even in the face of the most vile attacks. But Jenner never understood why his vaccination worked. In his time there was no theoretical ground for what he did. His achievement was the consequence of a simple, honest observation, true concern and common sense, all handled at their very best.

THE PROFESSIONAL RISKS for Jenner were high, but they were even higher for Pasteur. Jenner had begun his work with an observable fact: women in his area who had contracted cowpox did not seem to be able to contract smallpox. Pasteur began his work on sheer theory, on an overwhelming belief in science, and a sense of desperation. He was a chemist, not a physician. It was through his interest in organic chemistry and the problems of the French wine, beer, poultry and cattle industries that he became involved in medicine—a fact that even as he was curing the incurable, the medical profession never allowed him to forget. He would rather have remained with his first love, chemistry. It was there, toward the end of his life, that with all his medical achievements he felt he could still have done the most.

But Pasteur had the kind of mind that took him almost against his will from one investigation to another, from fermentations to infections and from there into the heart and guts of human disease and suffering. Throughout his life, he thought of others before himself. This humility did not spare him from the attacks of his contemporaries, chemists and physicians alike. In the course of a series of addresses defending his view that the cause of fermentation was spoilage produced by microorganisms, a sarcastic attack by one of his detractors, Pouquet, provoked him to actual wrath. Bitter, alone, he stood in front of the already hostile audience at the Academy of Sciences in Paris, and demanded that once and for all they stop the nonsense of their flowery speeches and keep their criticisms within the bounds of scientific thought and theory. He criticized the pompous etiquette of the Academy and its arrogant manner of procedure "that silenced the truth and stifled earnest creative thought." It was Paracelsus again and Harvey and Semmelweis. The medical establishment then did not like being scolded any more than in the time of Paracelsus or Semmelweis, and Pasteur paid the price for his courage the rest of his life. That the man who was destined to become the greatest medical figure of the nineteenth century was a chemist with no medical training at all shows how increasingly medicine, even though it refused to accept the situation, had come to rely on the rigorous application of the methods of physics and chemistry.

Pasteur's first discovery at the beginning of his scientific career was that chemical compounds giving the same chemical reactions and having the same physical properties could and did have different molecular configurations—different arrangements of the same identical atoms. This meant that their spatial arrangements—the three-dimensional configurations of compounds—though similar in every way could be as different as you and your image in the mirror. This early discovery, proved by using mixtures of racemic acid, paved the way for the whole new science of stereochemistry, the study of the physical arrangements of atoms inside of compounds.

Mitscherlich, one of the greatest scientists of the nineteenth century, had demonstrated in 1844 that two chemical compounds, the tartrates and the paratartrates of sodium and ammonia, had identical compositions—the same crystalline form, the same angles in their crystalline shape, the same double refraction, the same specific weights; in short, both were exactly the same. And yet, when they were dissolved in water, they caused a plane of a very special kind of light to rotate in exactly opposite directions. For years no one could explain this property. Among chemists it was a source of great discussion and even greater speculation.

The problem was finally solved by Pasteur working by himself, unsupported and unguided by any known fact or theory. Biot, a well-known chemist, was Pasteur's teacher at the time and had like other chemists been troubled over what had become known as Mitscherlich's planes. He knew that until the reason for the changing planes was discovered, a basic and perhaps fundamental property of organic substances would remain unsolved—a question which until answered could easily poison any new discovery. Mitscherlich's planes lay like a time bomb ready to go off in the face of any new chemical theory.

Pasteur's solving of the mystery was such an important event in Biot's life that years later his biographer could record precisely what had happened that day in his lab.

"Biot began by fetching some paratartaric acid. 'I have

most carefully studied it,' he said to Pasteur. 'It is absolutely neutral in the presence of polarized light.' Some distrust was visible in his gestures and audible in his voice. 'I shall bring you everything that is necessary,' he continued, fetching doses of soda and ammonia. He wanted this all prepared before his eyes. After pouring the liquid into a crystallizer Biot took it into a corner of his room to be quite sure that no one would touch it. 'I shall let you know when you are to come back,' he said to Pasteur.

"Forty-eight hours later some crystals, very small at first, began to form. When there was a sufficient number of them, Pasteur was recalled. Still in Biot's presence, Pasteur withdrew, one by one, the finest crystals and wiped off the mother liquid adhering to them. He then pointed out to Biot the opposition of their hemihedracal character—even though they were chemically and physically exactly alike—and divided them into two groups, left and right. 'So you affirm,' said Biot, 'that your right hand crystals would deviate the plane of polarization to the right, and your left hand ones will deviate to the left.' 'Yes,' said Pasteur.

" 'Well, let me do the rest.' Biot himself prepared the solutions and then sent again for Pasteur. Biot first placed in the polarized light apparatus a solution which should deviate to the left. Having satisfied himself that such a deviation actually took place, he took Pasteur's arm and said to him these words often deservedly quoted, 'My dear boy, I have loved science so much during my life that this touches my very heart.' "

"It was indeed evident," said Pasteur himself in recalling the event, "that the strongest light had been thrown on the cause of the phenomena of rotary polarization and hemihedral crystals; a new class of isomeric substances was discovered; the unexpected and until then unexampled constitution of the racemic or paratartaric acid was revealed." Pasteur's differentiation of the seemingly neutral racemic acid into the exactly identical right-handed and left-handed tartaric acids, which neutralize each other when the two acids are dissolved in water —combining in equal quantities—though still possessing equal and opposite rotatory powers because of different internal structures of the same atoms—was an extraordinary achievement. It is still considered to be, as written at the time, one of "the most daring attacks of the human mind upon unknown fields in chemistry."

It was the kind of approach that Pasteur was to bring to medicine. If past is prologue, nowhere is it more clearly shown than here in Pasteur's first great chemical discovery. The difficulty that all the other scientists had in solving the riddle of the Mitscherlich planes was quite simply the problem they had in trying to understand how two compounds could be different if everything about them was the same. Pasteur began his studies from the opposite direction. Freeing his mind of prejudices, he said to himself—perhaps even as a kind of numbed liturgy—that despite what everyone else said, despite all the chemical and physical conditions of the two substances being identical, there had to be a difference. These compounds simply could not be exactly the same in the face of the observable fact that their action on polarized light was so definitely opposite.

Pasteur's idea that there had to be a difference, his meticulousness in that idea's pursuit, his precise and honest application of rigorous scientific method as a tool to discovery helped him solve the riddle of the "planes" and was to carry him forward to become one of the greatest benefactors of mankind—and for most of his lifetime one of the most maligned of men. It was the discovery of the right- and left-handedness of organic substances that took him into the world of living things.

Why the dissymmetry? That was the obviously real scientific question and Pasteur pursued it. It soon became clear to him that all dissymmetrical compounds—those molecules alike in every way except that they rotated light either to the right or to the left—were all the products of living cells, whereas all mineral substances or compounds not formed from living organisms were symmetrical, were all left-handed. But why, again, this difference? Was the dissymmetry of organic compounds a fundamental distinction between life processes and nonorganic processes? Did life evolve from compounds that were only right-handed?

It was his study of the possible chemical differences between the living and nonliving that took Pasteur to the area of fermentation and from there to the study of animal pathology and finally to human disease itself. In studying the products of

fermentation, he discovered that fermentation was not the result of nonliving chemical substances called "ferments" getting
into foods and wines, which was the accepted theory, but the
result of living organisms, microbes, using the fermentable substances for their own metabolism and in the process changing
the fermentable substances, like wine into vinegar. Pasteur presented his new theory and its indisputable supportive data,
proving the microbial basis of fermentation, to the Academy of
Sciences. The idea of living substances causing chemical
changes was in direct opposition to the accepted theories of
"ferments" as well as the then accepted theory of "spontaneous
generation."

It is hard to know on which challenge he was attacked more
violently—that there were no "ferments" or that there was no
such thing as "spontaneous generation," that living things did
not simply appear in spoiled food and drink or decaying
material. The enmity that was to follow him all his life began
here in his attacks on these accepted and honored theories. But
in 1867, using his new theory, he single-handedly saved the wine
industry of France by proving that the spoilage of wine was
indeed caused by microorganisms and that the spoilage could
be prevented by partial heat sterilization at 55 to 60 degrees
Centigrade (130 to 140 degrees F.) without changing the taste of
the vintage. This is the process we now call pasteurization.
Using the same methods and his same theory, Pasteur went on
to save the beer industry. Step by step, having to establish one
fact before he could proceed to the next, running into dead ends
and having to begin again, he had proved himself and his theories right.

Yet through all these years of rescuing French industry he
was attacked almost gleefully for the slowness of his progress
and for his seeming inability to really and conclusively disprove
the theory of spontaneous generation. Pasteur prevailed, although at great cost to himself. It was during this time of repeated personal and professional attacks that he suffered a
stroke, his daughter died, and economics became a burden.

With one final classic experiment he put to rest once and
for all the idea of spontaneous generation and at the same time
the concept of "ferments." Devising a hollow dumbbell-shaped
flask, he placed some sterilized meat in one end of the flask and

a culture of bacteria in the other end, with a trap in the thin hollowed portion between them, Pasteur showed that no matter what was done to the meat and for how long, spoilage occurred only if the trap between the two portions of the flask was removed and the bacteria allowed to reach the meat.

His fame grew, and while the professionals continued their criticism, the public turned in increasing numbers to him, at first to protect their livelihoods and then eventually to protect their lives.

In the late eighteen hundreds the chicken industry in France was being decimated by the disease of cholera. Pasteur was asked to help. He agreed, and two years later after almost nothing but solid backbreaking work, he isolated the bacteria that he was sure caused the epidemic. He collected the diarrheal feces from the diseased birds, cultured it, tediously and meticulously isolated the organism; then, using Koch's culture mediums, he began growing these organisms in pure culture. Eventually the bacteria growing in the test tubes became so thick that they outgrew the nutrients on which they fed and began to die, so that Pasteur had to continually transfer a few healthy colonies to ever newer flasks to keep the strains alive. One day by mistake he took an old culture that had been growing for weeks and injected the contents into young healthy birds. They did not get the disease. Again, here was an observable fact—with no available explanation. He took other old cultures and tried again and the birds did not get cholera.

There is a reason; "trust in science," he'd said. With the thought comforting him he pursued the answer, and in that pursuit did an extraordinary thing: he took bacteria from a new culture, injected part into the healthy birds and part into birds that he had given the old culture. Why he did this no one knows, but it was to prove one of the most fortunate acts of all time. The birds that had previously been injected with the old culture remained healthy even when given the new deadly culture; those that had not been given the old culture died as expected. The only explanation available was that somehow the cholera bacteria in the old culture had become "weakened," so that injected into the healthy chickens, they did not cause disease; somehow the "weakened" or dead bacteria had managed to protect the chickens from their next exposure to the normal healthy cholera-causing bacteria. The real questions now were: What had weakened the bacteria? What was the nature of the protection?

Pasteur presented his new discovery. It was taken up by the farmers, and although he had saved the chicken industry, his detractors declared there must have been some material in the older cultures he injected, along with the dead and dying bacteria, that protected the chickens. Pasteur knew that the only things in that culture were the bacteria and the innocuous nutrient medium itself. The answer, he was sure, was a whole new theory: the bacteria that caused the cholera were "weakened" or killed by continually growing in the broth which had with age become deficient, and these dead or weakened bacteria in some way had caused the protection. He took the idea one step further. Perhaps, he reasoned, what he had discovered with the chicken cholera bacteria was a general phenomenon, that any microbe causing disease could be "weakened" by passing it through successive generations in places other than where it would normally grow—an artificial culture medium or an animal that it usually did not infect.

At the time, anthrax was ravaging the animal herds of France. The sheep and cattle men, like the chicken farmers before them, came to Pasteur. Koch's discovery of the anthrax bacillus had done nothing to stop the disease. But again using Koch's discovery, Pasteur obtained and isolated the anthrax bacillus. Growing the bacteria in cultures, collecting millions of them, he then tried another experiment; he simply killed them with phenol and injected the killed bacteria into sheep. As with the injections of the "weakened" cholera bacillus, injections of the dead anthrax worked, too—none of the injected animals acquired the disease. It was the first widely used bacterial killed vaccine, and with it Pasteur saved the sheep and cattle herds of Europe.

WHATEVER IT IS that leads to genius, whatever its cause— chance, hard work, refusal to accept limitations, understanding of the tools at hand and what can truly be done with them, or simply a feeling, an unexplainable sense that guides when there

are no signposts; courage, daring, foolishness, or just not knowing any other way; all or pieces of them all—whatever it was,
Pasteur had it. He was an authentic genius.

The idea of manipulating disease—changing the disease-
causing organisms so that they would protect the host from the
disease-causing microbe—was a new concept. For the first time
in the history of mankind Pasteur applied his new concept to
the curing of a human disease—rabies. In 1878 he took up the
challenge that drove him so far ahead of any physician who had
ever lived there would have been no place for him to hide had
he failed.

Of all the scourges of man the one that was most feared and
most deadly, that was 100 percent fatal, was rabies. No one ever
bitten by a rabid dog was ever spared, no one. Its lethality, the
terror and hopelessness of those bitten, were known to Pasteur.
But perhaps, he thought, there was a way out. Turning his
attention to this plague, he used what he had already learned,
and leaving more and more of his beloved chemistry behind, he
reported in 1881 that rabies was not caused by bacteria but by
a filterable material which he had found in the saliva of rabid
animals. What it was, he didn't know. All he was sure of was that
it was not bacterial, but was nevertheless infectious.

Year by year, with the same tenacity he had attacked all
other problems, by then half paralyzed by his stroke, Pasteur
kept after this question. He found the infectious material in the
brains of animals after he injected them with rabid saliva. How
did it get there? He then found the material in the peripheral
nerves of the animals and discovered that it traveled from the
area of injection up those nerves to the brain. He discovered
that it took weeks for the substance—whatever it was—using
this route to reach the animal's brain cells, where it caused
madness and finally death. This was the reason, he postulated,
that there was always the gap between the time an animal was
bitten and the time he began to have seizures and go insane.
Pasteur proved his theory by finding he could produce rabies
more quickly in experimental animals by injecting the saliva of
rabid dogs into areas progressively closer to the animal's brain
—the face, head and neck—and most quickly by injecting it
directly into the brain itself.

Applying the methods he had discovered for chicken chol-

era and for anthrax, he "weakened" the substance by injecting
it into the animals of another species, removing their diseased
brains, then drying the tissue and using it as a vaccine. He
injected some dogs with the "weakened" material grown in
rabbits, then put them in with other animals that were not
inoculated and turned a rabid dog loose among them. All were
bitten and all the unprotected dogs died. Here finally was a way
to cure rabies, and Pasteur suggested that all the dogs in France
be vaccinated.

Since he was not a physician, he never thought of using the
vaccine on humans. But news of the vaccine had spread, and in
1885 a desperate mother, without concern for protocol, brought
her son to Pasteur in his laboratory in Alsace and begged him
for help. Her son, a nine-year-old shepherd boy, had been bitten
by a rabid dog. Pasteur responded to the pleas of the distraught
mother, and putting aside his reluctance to encroach on the
territory of the physicians, examined the boy and found fourteen bites on the child's hands and arms. He had already proved
that the cause of rabies, whatever it was, reached the brain by
the slow movement up the nerves, beginning at the place of the
bite. Perhaps by injecting the new vaccine, there might still be
time to protect the child.

But in his experiments with dogs Pasteur had immunized
them *before* they were bitten, and this boy was already infected. Would the vaccine work in time? What if the dog that
had bitten him was not rabid, but simply crazy or ill from another disease, like a brain tumor or meningitis? Would the vaccine with his "weakened" but still infectious material kill the
boy? He could wait until the child showed signs of the rabies,
but by then it would already be in the boy's brain, and it would
certainly be too late. If there was any hope at all, the material
had to be stopped—neutralized—before it reached the brain.

Pasteur had no place to turn. There was no one else in the
world who knew more than he did about rabies, but there were
many who were willing to criticize. "Human experimenta-
tions!" they cried. "You are not a physician." The medical establishment warned of treatment without a medical license. The
law-enforcement agencies, prodded by the medical profession,
also warned of prosecution. But there were some physicians
who, realizing the hopelessness of the situation, counseled him

that the vaccine with all its possible limitations was the only hope.

Pasteur agreed and began the injections. The world waited, enemies waited, and a little boy and his mother waited.

"I could not sleep the night before the last injection," Pasteur wrote. "The material I was using was so deadly, so undiluted that it killed an unprotected rabbit in less than a day." It worked, though. But how? A new era of medicine had opened and the struggle to find the answer to that question was to become the next great battleground of medicine.

5

Our Immune System: Early Discoveries

EVERY LIVING ORGANISM has to defend itself. The struggle for food in the eat-or-be-eaten world that evolved out of those first seas had made protection a crucial factor in survival.

We can best understand what our immune system means, what has to be given us in order to survive, by looking at diseases in other living things—plants.

Bacteria and viruses and fungi cause diseases in plants as well as in humans and animals. The tobacco mosaic virus, for example, infects the tobacco plant, but unlike other microbes that attack the roots or stems, the tobacco mosaic virus attacks primarily the plant's leaves, multiplying in the leaves' green cells, killing the chloroplasts, which make the plant's chlorophyll. The virus spreads a little each day. As with all plant infections, the spread is slow; one leaf dies as another begins. Illness in plants is, for the most part, a localized process. With virtually no circulation, there is no rapid spread of infecting microbes, no quick movement of contagion from one place to another, no overall consumption; unlike animals and humans, there is no half-day of listlessness and the next day death. A diseased leaf or root may eventually decay, but the rest of the plant will live on, unconcernedly giving up the diseased part as it grows a new one, forming new leaves and roots even as the old ones decay and die. It is not that the microbes which attack plants are less powerful or destructive than those which attack us, or that they are any less ruthless; they simply cannot move through the plant as rapidly as they can move through us, and that slowness is in reality the plant's major protection.

We humans do not have the luxury of time. The total blood volume in our body circulates once every thirteen seconds; sixty quarts of blood pass to the brain and the kidneys per hour, and it is all returned to the heart at the same rate. The volumes moved are tremendous and it is these volumes that give us the ability to run, to keep enough oxygen and sugar moving to our legs and arms so that our muscles can move even after hours of exertion.

Every cell of our body lies within the drifts and tides of our circulation. Unlike the early seas, where the oxygen and sugars, the proteins and fats that were necessary for cells to function reached them through the uncertain wash of the ocean waters, or as in the beginnings of evolution, through the slow sluggish movements of primitive circulations, our cells are supplied by a regular high-pressure system delivering, whenever necessary, vast amounts of raw materials, of oxygen and sugars, so that these cells can function optimally and for long periods of time. Under stress, our heart, pounding at the rate of 200 or 250 times a minute, can move incredible amounts of materials to and from struggling cells. The fuels will continue to be brought, washing past each of the body's cells, keeping them working long beyond what any of us consider even human endurance, long beyond what any cell could have done in the whole long history of evolution. This cellular ability to function at sustained gigantic rates is given to us by the circulatory system; it ensures our mobility, strength, speed and agility. It has given us our chance to flee or to fight, to exist, to endure, to win.

But the price paid for all this quickness as well as power is a severe one. A bacterium from a cut in your finger can reach your brain in a little over four seconds. A pneumococcus in your lungs can reach the bones of your arms in three seconds. A meningococcus lodging in your nose or throat could be in the meninges of your brain in ten seconds. The tobacco mosaic virus —indeed, any virus or bacterium that attacks plants—upon entering our body, would be in every one of our organs within minutes. It would be growing in our kidneys, heart and lungs, in our bones, spleen and liver, our brain and our muscles, killing us before we even felt the first waves of illness.

The evolutionary demands and requirements to ensure our protection with a circulatory system such as we have are so overwhelming it is numbing to think of what is involved. Yet, astonishingly, the protection is there. It is the end result of a thousand million years of finely honed chemical responsiveness: a group of chemical protectors and microbial killers so quick and so vicious that despite our size, our circulatory system, all our human mistakes, misdeeds and blunders, we survive.

For decades after the discovery of the smallpox and rabies vaccines, men spent their lives and some their fortunes trying to understand how and why vaccinations worked. From Pasteur on, the greatest efforts in scientific medicine were devoted to uncovering the remarkable events occurring in the bodies of people and animals who had been immunized. Physicians realized early that in understanding how vaccines worked, they would not only know how to protect people but how each of us maintains his health and how we become ill. At first they approached the problem in bits and pieces, not quite knowing what they were doing and even at times what they were looking for. Using inadequate equipment and dealing with the crudest preparations, they managed somehow through the years to put together the answers.

Metchnikoff, beginning in Pasteur's laboratory in 1888, worked most of his adult life to prove that the special white cells he found in the blood of animals and humans, cells loaded with strange, darkly staining granules, increase in number during bacterial infections, and protect us by eating the infecting bacteria. These granulocytes are the same white cells your family doctor measures today when he does a white count of your blood, knowing that if there is an infection anywhere in your body, there will be an increased number of them in your circulation.

Metchnikoff's discovery that we have within us circulating

white cells which protect us from bacterial invasion by eating bacteria was the beginning of our understanding of the immune system.

In the last decade of that century Von Behring proved that when a person is infected with diphtheria, he develops a substance in his blood which neutralizes the toxin of that infecting organism. He called this neutralizing substance antitoxin, and went on to show how diphtheria could be treated by injecting the antitoxin into the infected person.

In those same years Pfeiffer, painstakingly using his microscope, made the astonishing discovery that bacteria injected into the body were destroyed intravascularly and that this destruction had nothing to do with Metchnikoff's granulocytes. He actually saw the bacteria, once in the animal's bloodstream, swell up and then, as if suddenly detonated, blow apart. Precisely what it was in the serum of blood that destroyed bacteria as well as neutralized diphtheria toxin, it would take another half-century to find out.

But it was a beginning. By the turn of the century, scientists at least knew there were two parts to our immune system: a cellular defense made up of Metchnikoff's granulocytes, and a serum defense made up of specifically manufactured, though then unknown blood factors. Work continued simultaneously on the unraveling of these two parts of the system.

It was soon discovered that the granulocytes of immunized animals attacked and killed bacteria more quickly than did those of nonimmunized animals. Shortly after that discovery it was found that the blood from immunized subjects could by itself, without any white cells, clump together injected bacteria, while nonimmunized blood could not. Clearly, immunization did something to both parts of the immune system, to the white cells of the immunized animal and to its serum factors.

Today we can repeat those early experiments. We can take blood from a nonimmunized animal, put it in a petri dish filled with live bacteria, and watch under the microscope how the granulocytes move around, come up against the bacteria and try to engulf them, while the bacteria just slide away and continue even in the presence of the granulocytes to grow and divide. But immunize the animal first with the same bacteria and then take its blood and put it into the shallow dish with the same bacteria used for the injections, and the whole picture changes. The bacteria suddenly stick together and the granulocytes in the drop of blood move right in after them; there is no slipping away now. The granulocytes barely seem to brush up against the bacteria, and the microbes are swallowed. Within minutes there are no bacteria left alive in the dish. Under the microscope you can actually see them inside the granulocytes, being slowly digested by the white cells' granules.

Less than a hundred years ago Koch performed an experiment whose results stunned everyone and that only now we are truly beginning to understand. He injected a large dose of tuberculin—a protein he had extracted chemically from the cell walls of the bacillus that causes tuberculosis—into the bodies of already tuberculous guinea pigs. Within three hours the guinea pigs became ill, and in less than sixteen they were all dead, killed by nothing more than an injection of a part of the tuberculous bacilli. There could have been no possible additional infection because no live bacteria were used, only a portion of their cell walls. Yet, obviously something catastrophic had happened in these injected animals.

When Koch next injected the tuberculin just into the skin of tuberculous animals, nothing happened—at least at first. But within six hours the site of the injection began to blanch and then to swell; the whole area became red and inflamed. When the tissue was examined under the microscope, the swollen, inflamed and dying skin was found to be filled from top to bottom not with granulocytes, but with another kind of white cell: small, lightly staining lymphocytes, white cells similar to Metchnikoff's granulocytes but without their darkly staining granules.

These white cells had always been noticed on microscopic blood smears side by side with the granulocytes, but had been ignored. Now, all of a sudden, they were found by the thousands in areas of damaged and dying tissue, damage caused by the injection of merely parts of the tubercule bacillus.

A new cell had been added to our recognition of the body's defenses. Nobody knew what it did, but by the nineteen-tens it was plain that our immune system was made up not of two, but of three parts: the circulating granulocytes, the serum factors, and now the circulating lymphocytes.

[6 3]

The same thing that had happened with Koch's experimental animals occurred when the skins of humans suffering and dying from tuberculosis were injected with tuberculin. Lymphocytes flooded into the injection sites, and the same swelling, redness and tissue destruction took place in the human skin that had occurred in the skin of the tuberculous guinea pigs. Again it was observed under the microscope that the inflamed areas, out to the very margins of the inflammation and tissue destruction, were completely filled with these immunologic cells.

Unexplainable discoveries were made, too, concerning the other parts of immunity. In the early nineteen hundreds two researchers, Richet and Portier, pursuing the serum-factor part of our immune system, had rediscovered and extended the experiments of Magendie that had been done seventy years before. At that time Magendie, the greatest European physiologist of his day, had shown that dogs previously injected intravenously with proteins from other animals would experience a severe and fatal reaction if ever injected a second time. Neither he nor anyone else at the time appreciated the significance of his observations and its relationship both to how we fight infections and to what would eventually be called allergy.

Using Magendie's methods, the two researchers demonstrated that certain dogs could survive an initial dose of protein toxin, but unlike those injected with the toxins of diphtheria, or even the cholera or anthrax bacillus, these animals failed to show immunity to a second injection, and in fact died within minutes.

Richet and Portier went on to show that even if you injected something as innocuous as the white of an egg into animals, and followed this in another week or so with another dose of egg whites, these animals would be dead within minutes of the second injection. Not only that, but strange and unexplainable substances had developed in the blood of these animals. New serum factors not there before the second injection were found that would, after the animals' death, combine in test tubes with the egg whites similar to those used in the injections, causing the egg whites to clump together and fall to the bottom of the tube. Apparently, to everyone's surprise, immunization could be as dangerous as it was helpful.

In all the confusion of trying to understand what was happening, scientists championed their own favorite theories. Some said immunity had to do solely with the person's granulocytes, others held it was the serum factors. A few talked only of allergy, others only of protection. Theses were developed maintaining that the clumping of the bacteria was critical to our protection, while still other propositions stated that it was the intravascular detonation and destruction of the microbes that sustained us.

The confusion gradually cleared. People suffering from viral illnesses or worm infections were found to have increased lymphocytes in their bloodstream, not increased granulocytes. It was noticed that in cases of skin eruption caused by poison ivy or poison oak, the reaction in the skin followed the same delayed time course as in those animals injected with tuberculin, and that the skin of these lesions showed the same swelling and in severe cases exactly the same ulceration, and contained the same lymphocytes, as were seen in the tuberculin skin reactions.

Finally, in 1925, Zinsser showed what no one had suspected —that everybody was right, that defense against bacterial or viral invasion was simply too important for the body to leave to any one system and therefore it employed several: the cellular system made up of the various kinds of white cells, the granulocytes and lymphocytes, and the humoral system made up of a combination of different but very special serum factors. Zinsser proved that all the bodily reactions against infection involve the three parts of the immune system working together, and that one or the other predominates depending on the kind of infection or the type of material injected.

But it was not until 1937 that scientists were finally able to establish exactly what the serum factors involved in the immune response were, how they clumped and destroyed bacteria and also helped the granulocytes and lymphocytes do their killing. This discovery opened up the modern age of immunology, and with it not only an understanding of how immunization works but also a real understanding of allergy, and why injections of some foreign substances, if given a second time, could lead to death.

In that year Tiselius devised a method of using electricity to separate blood proteins one from the other. He took blood samples from human volunteers, and putting the samples on gelatin discs, applied an electric charge across the gel. What Tiselius had discovered, what led to the development of his electrophoretic machine, was the fact that the proteins in the blood, comprised as they all are of atoms of carbon, hydrogen, oxygen and nitrogen, are electrically charged, and depending on the numbers and kinds of atoms that make up their molecular structure, they each have a different total electric charge. Attracted or repelled by the positive or negative charges at the edges of the electric field, the proteins would migrate through the gel at different rates depending on their total charges.

The more positively charged proteins would move faster toward the negative pole of the machine than those more negatively charged. Electrophoresis was a process that took advantage of nothing more than the different physical electrical characteristics of proteins, characteristics that had been there since those proteins were first formed billions of years ago, and were now, through one man's ingenuity, used to separate them, to physically distinguish one from another. Tiselius found there were three different groups of proteins in human blood, the three groups migrating at different rates. He called the first the alpha globulins, because they were the proteins that moved fastest through the gel and so were the closest to the negative pole of his machine. The second he called the beta globulins, and the third the gamma globulins.

Actually his method of separation was very crude; it was like dividing all moving vehicles into those that move on rails, those that move on wheels, and those that move on treads. Within each group there were still many different kinds of proteins. You can have a streetcar or a freight train moving on tracks, and a tricycle or an automobile moving on wheels. But crude as his method was, by taking advantage of a fundamental difference of proteins—their differing electric charge—an astonishingly important discovery was made: the serum factors in the blood that helped granulocytes to devour microbes, that neutralized diphtheria toxins and caused bacteria to clump together, were all in the protein fraction of the blood that he had called the gamma globulins. There was none of this kind of immunologic activity in the alpha or beta blood-protein fractions. These serum factors, all proteins migrating in the gamma-globulin fraction of human blood, were given the name "antibodies" because they were the blood proteins produced in response to bodily attacks by foreign substances.

Tiselius' discovery gave immunologists the tool they had been looking for since Pasteur. They could finally separate antibodies from all other proteins in the blood, concentrate them and have purified material to work with.

In 1948 Fagraeus proved that antibodies are produced by special cells in the body's bone marrow and lymph nodes, cells which he called plasma cells. It was later found that these plasma cells themselves came from the lymphocytes. But it was not until 1962, less than fifteen years ago and a full three quarters of a century after Pasteur's death, that scientists truly began to understand precisely what antibodies are, what they are made of, how they work, how they help granulocytes kill bacteria, how they clump bacteria and how they interact with lymphocytes.

So important has this work been to our understanding of disease and illness as well as health that three Nobel prizes have already been given for the discoveries, and in the next two decades five or ten more probably will be awarded.

What follows deals with the fruits of these labors, with what goes on inside of us and for us every moment of every day of our lives, what is going on in your own body right now, silently, relentlessly, even as you read these words.

6

Our Immune System:
The Protectors

IN EARTHWORMS and some octopuses, the earliest beginnings of truly integrated multicellular animal life, we find for the first time a primitive circulation. And in that circulation we find a still more primitive kind of cell.

It is a cell so totally different from the other, more specialized cells in these early animals' bodies that it is almost as if it might have swum in one day and just decided to stay, or more probably, that unlike the other cells, it refused to progress, to become more specialized, retaining its original movability and independence. The evolutionary advantage to these early animals of having such primitive cells a part of themselves is obvious, so much so that today it is hard to know whether the amoeboid cells moving through these animals' tissues are the result of their circulation or whether they allowed that circulation to develop.

Under the microscope the cells can be seen moving slowly, searchingly, through the earthworm's body, slipping past the cells of its gut and muscles, creeping along the two or three layers of tissue planes, shifting their movement, insinuating themselves into and out of the newly formed circulatory channels, constantly picking up bits and pieces of cellular debris and ingesting them. In one sense, these primitive phagocytic cells act as an internal garbage system. But they also serve another function; they will fight. They will attack any bacterium they meet, throw themselves against it in a struggle older than life, and keep at it until one or the other is dead. And in fact, half the time these cells lose. Partly it is because they are not really all that good at fighting, and partly because some of the bacteria they come up against have evolved far beyond them, developing through the ages of their own evolution protective capsules and elaborate poisons that give them the edge. Or they lose because there are just too many bacteria for them to handle successfully. But as ineffectual as these primitive cells sometimes are, as chancy as their interception of an infecting bacterium may be and as unequal the fight, they are there, and just by being there, give the earthworm with its slow circulation and all its more specialized cells—immobile, unprotected, open to attack—a means of internal defense, the evolutionary edge that allowed life to continue to evolve.

It is these primitive cells that we have inherited. Their descendants are the Metchnikoff white cells, the granulocytes, which are more specialized today than when they appeared in the first earthworms; they have evolved along with us and are now better fitted to kill bacteria. In the millions of years of evolving along with us, the granulocytes have become more vicious and more mobile, and have acquired a whole new arsenal of bacterial inhibitors and poisons, stored in their darkly staining granules. They are able now to phagocytize more quickly and even able to move toward the microbes rather than just wait for them to come by, or happen on them by chance. Our granulocytes can even sense where they are and where they must go, and there are now not merely a few available to us, but literally billions. These white cells, and an even more specialized version, the macrophages, are all made in our bone marrow, mature there and are then released into the bloodstream ready to fight. A few are always on patrol in our vessels, but the rest are available in case of attack. The average 150-pound man or woman has 126 billion granulocytes and macrophages available. The body can, on command, release them all, and sometimes all are needed.

Pus, the sticky yellowish blood-tinged material that oozes out of infected wounds and out of abscesses, is an indicator of the unending battle and constant bitterness of the struggle. The pus contains not only dead bacteria but dead and dying granulocytes, at times millions of both. In an area of an infection, both granulocytes and bacteria are killing and being killed. It is not a very subtle battle; there is no death at a distance here. The granulocytes, coming into physical contact with the bacterium, try to engulf it, to corner and finally murder it. And the bacterium, elaborating poisons, moving this way and that, protected by its walls and polysaccharide capsule, tries to kill the granulocytes before it is killed itself.

With all their new-found evolutionary sophistication, their greater mobility, more powerful digestive enzymes and more potent killing abilities, each granulocyte still wins by having retained the primitive savagery of its remote ancestors. Its attack today is a mixture of ancient ruthlessness coupled with modern chemical sophistication. If you take a syringe and withdraw 10 cc. of blood from your arm, separate out the granulocytes and place them in a small dish filled with salt water, they will move about randomly. Under the microscope they crawl like tiny amoebas this way and that. It is a rather tranquil picture, reminiscent of types of algae-like organisms moving slowly along the shoreline. All you have to do is add one bacterium to the dish, just one, and the whole scene changes. The dish suddenly becomes another world. The granulocytes, like alerted deer, suddenly stop their random movements; a certain expectancy and wariness seems to grip them. Hesitatingly, almost nervously at first, they move this way and that, as if sensing something, and then, all of a sudden, they move off, one by one, in the direction of the bacterium, creeping slowly, relentlessly toward the microbe.

In the body this movement carries the granulocytes out of the blood vessels toward the place of infection. It is the first movement in an assault by a 126-billion-man army. So effective is this internal sonar that within minutes of the beginning of an infection, the first of the granulocytes are already in the area, attacking the bacteria. Once started, they fight so determinedly, expend so much energy, that once committed, they can exist in the battle for at best only a short time. But by then their bigger brothers, the macrophages—which look much like granulocytes but are larger and more sophisticated cells with greater amounts of killing enzymes, greater endurance, thicker membranes and larger internal machineries—arrive and take over the attack. Despite their huge numbers, the granulocytes are really shock troops. As with any agile attack force, their greater mobility has been paid for by lighter armaments and restricted energy stores.

Once the bigger, tougher macrophages establish themselves in the infected area, the granulocytes back off and let the macrophages make the fight alone. It is an extraordinary sequence of events, but it comes about because of one simple ageless fact: once provoked, these white cells will attack without the slightest hesitation. They will attack any foreign substance and keep after it until one or both are destroyed. You can take a drop of pus and under the microscope see these white cells fighting for our lives. You can actually see them grab the bacteria and hold them while they empty their granules onto them; you can see the microbes twist and turn, gradually cease their movements, and begin finally to break apart. Even after infections you can still see some of these white cells, beaten and worn, back in the circulation with bits and pieces of microbial cell walls still inside them, again moving slowly through the bloodstream, continuing their unending patrols, and ready, even battered and wounded, for the next battle.

THE GRANULOCYTES and macrophages in our bloodstream are only part of our immune system. Indeed, if they were all we had, we would not survive very long. Those children born with combined immunodeficiency have all the granulocytes they need, yet they die within months from infections. By themselves granulocytes aren't fast enough; with bacterial infections even a few minutes is too long. Once through the skin and into the bloodstream, a bacterium would be on its way to the brain or lungs long before the first granulocyte could possibly reach it. We need more, and we have it. Life is too precious to have been left with only one system of defense. Very early in the nineteenth century, physiologists studying the body realized that the more important to survival the process they were studying, the more backup systems the body had developed to make sure that that process would keep going.

We have not one way of maintaining our blood pressure but four; there is not one system for keeping our tissue fluids at the correct acidity but seven. It is the same with our defenses. The parts, humoral and cellular, may seem independent but each one aids the other, giving us a total defense truly greater than any of its parts. The necessity for this interaction becomes obvious when the granulocyte reaches an infected area. It is suddenly faced with a confusing array of different chemical products and various types of cellular debris—not only bacteria but leaking cells and thrombin plugs, fragmented blood proteins, fats, denatured enzymes, broken-up membranes—the rubble of the battle. Yet it can't waste itself on anything but the bacterium, nor, once it gets close, can it afford to let the enemy slip away from it. It is the second part of our defense system, our antibodies, which make sure that granulocytes do their job as well as they can. They coat the bacterium, and at the same time they help direct the granulocyte toward it, through all the press of cellular debris.

Most of what we know about antibodies has been learned only in the last ten years. We know now that they are really nothing more than special proteins circulating in our bloodstream. Our blood is a high-speed expressway delivering fats and sugars, fatty acids, hormones, minerals, salt and water to all parts of the body, while at the same time carrying away wastes. Proteins, too, are moved along this expressway.

Proteins made up of linked-together amino acids are structurally solid compounds, very stable. And since the amino acids that form proteins can be linked to form protein molecules of almost any length and three-dimensional structure, proteins become eminently suited to be the structural building blocks of the body. And they are. They make up our skin and muscle fibers, our ligaments and tendons, our hair and nails. Because of their unique chemical stability and internal strength, they act as messengers, the hormones and the enzymes carrying information from one place in the body to another. Proteins have another ability besides structural soundness; since they can be added to, they can be made to fit around almost any "foreign" structure.

When this first happened, we don't know. Proteins have been a part of life from its very beginning. Indeed, because of their linkage ability they were in all probability the first polymers. But when exactly a cell first used its proteins to couple with the surface of a different cell, when it first turned a protein into an antibody we don't know. It appears to have occurred in the most primitive group of living vertebrates, the jawless fishes. Swimming about in the warm, teeming Paleozoic seas, there must have occurred a mutation, a chance event. A protein, used by those hagfishes and lampreys for some other purpose, maybe even as an enzyme controlling some cellular metabolic event, must suddenly have mutated, changed its structure and was then able to attach itself to part of the surfaces of foreign particles that entered these fishes' bodies.

Like the more primitive earthworm, the jawless fishes had the ancestors of our granulocytes within them. The amoeboid cells patrolled their vessels and organs, as they did the lower earthworm's, but now there was something else—a protein that could fix to the attacker and hold it, perhaps even interrupt its own defenses. The primitive granulocyte was no longer on its own. It now had help.

The lampreys and hagfishes are still with us, unchanged in almost 600 million years. We can take them today into the laboratory and see in them our own immunologic beginnings. If you take skin from another species and graft it onto these fishes, they will, like ourselves, reject the graft. But while we reject it in a few days, the lampreys and hagfishes barely begin to reject theirs even after two months.

We find in their blood primitive antibodies that have some ability to combine with the surfaces of certain foreign materials. For all that our own more sophisticated antibodies do, their function remains essentially the same as what those primitive antibodies do for the hagfish. What that is can be seen in any medical laboratory in the world. Take some blood from a hagfish or lamprey, separate out the blood proteins and mix it in a test tube with your own blood. Hold the test tube up to the light, and you will soon see the red cells in your blood begin to clump together and slowly drift down to the bottom of the test tube.

It is not a very spectacular event. There is no light, no heat given off, there is not even any foaming or turbulence. Watching those red cells clump and fall slowly to the bottom of the test tube has all the excitement of watching a piece of ice gradually melt. But it is just as relentless a process, and for all its lack of splendor, it is in reality the difference between life and death. It is why we survive our wound infections, and our children their flus and pneumonias, why 50 percent and not 100 percent of women with puerperal fever died and why less than one percent of children with measles become brain-damaged. It is the reason why our bladder infections get better and our boils gradually go away.

The antibodies in the hagfish's blood attach themselves to our red blood cells and clump them together, and the heavy clumps fall to the bottom of the test tube. In the hundreds of millions of years of evolution from the hagfish to us, this ability of proteins to clump together foreign substances has been modified and refined, tuned and heightened into an antibody system of defense which is so chemically sophisticated and powerful that for all the modern tools of medical science, we are only now beginning to understand how incredibly complex the system is, how powerful it has become.

Our body, unlike the hagfish's, manufactures not one kind of antibody but three. All are proteins, all migrate electrophoretically as gamma globulins, and all evolved from that first hagfish antibody. But they differ now one from the other and from the original antibody in size, amino-acid sequence, and most important, the place in the body where they do their attacking.

First there is the antibody called IgA (for Immunoglobulin A), which is secreted in our tears and saliva; it is present in all the secretions that coat our gastrointestinal tract, the saliva of our mouth and throat, the secretions of our stomach, intestines and rectum. Our skin itself acts as a formidable barrier against infection, a defense against microbes. Its thickness and scaliness keep out all attackers. But our other coverings are not so impervious; the mucous membranes that line our lips, the soft covering of our eyes, the inside of our nose and cheeks, the linings of our mouth, throat and stomach are all as open to the outside as our skin, but without the skin's scaly protection. To keep organisms from entering through these moist, open surfaces, our body in its evolutionary wisdom coats them with IgA antibodies, literally pumps them out in the secretions that bathe all these internal surfaces, so that the linings are always covered with a few hundred or a few thousand of these antibody molecules. As long as the area is kept moist, the antibodies will attack any microbe, couple with any bacterium, fungus or virus that comes their way, clumping them, slowing them down, stopping them from getting through the linings into the bloodstream or down into the deeper layers of our bodies.

But even with the outer defenses of our skin, and the IgA-coated mucous membranes, we can still be infected. The skin can be cut, the membranes can be breached. Of the million streptococci that might attack our throat, one can escape the IgA molecules and get through into our circulation. This has plainly happened enough times in evolution for our bodies to make two other antibodies, called IgG (for Immunoglobulin G) and IgM (for Immunoglobulin M), both of which circulate in our bloodstream. The IgM antibody is larger, less mobile than the IgG, and in a sense it is much more determined.

We should have learned by now to trust the body, but we haven't. For years immunologists wondered at the foolishness of having two antibodies in our circulation, both doing exactly the same thing, traveling side by side, differing only in size. Our body, not foolish and never wasteful, has a reason: the protection of our young.

All children are born with a limited ability to make antibodies. Time is the absolute requirement to bring their antibodies up to protective circulatory levels. Antibodies do not simply or magically appear in our children's bodies; they are produced, and it is how they are produced that is one of the major evolutionary achievements. A mixture of mystery and chemistry, it is a combination of physics and grace down at the molecular level, where despite our sense of importance and dominance, our lives are still preciously maintained.

Life is still what it always has been, a battle of molecules, of our chemistry against the invaders'.

•   •   •

ANTIBODIES are manufactured by cells in our body in response to what those cells determine are foreign markers on the surface of the attacking microbes. These markers are molecular configurations in the membranes of the invaders, or in the structures of materials. They make configurations which differ from the arrangement of the molecules in the membranes of our body's own cells and in the materials we make for ourselves. We call these different markers "antigens," and it is against the antigens on a foreign cell's surface or an injected toxin that antibodies are made.

The astonishing fact is that the antibody-producing cells of our body not only know what is their own but everything that is foreign, or probably more accurately, everything that is not "theirs." The enormity of that task is simply stunning.

Our body is constantly breaking down. Bits and pieces of it are always entering the circulation: membranes from aging red cells, parts of broken-down hormones and enzymes, leaky tissues, dying cells. It is constantly being filled with cellular debris, not only normal fragments but distorted pieces mauled by usage and seemingly beyond any chemical recognition. In cases of infection it is even worse; the distortions in altered proteins and the chemical changes in the infected and dying cells become even greater. Yet amid all this confusion the cells that produce our antibodies, our plasma cells, can distinguish what is normal and what is not. They can pick out the foreign particles, the microbes, the poisons, and using the antigens on their surface make the antibodies which, when released into the circulation, will fit exactly the antigens on the attackers' surface, atom for atom, and molecule for molecule.

Never the aggressor, doomed always to have to react, to be forever the counterattacker, the body must first have the microbes or poisons already inside it before it can begin to manufacture the appropriate IgG and IgM antibodies. That is the greatest weakness in our whole antibody system. In a constant state of paranoia, the body is forever at a disadvantage; always behind at the beginning, it must gather its forces and go after an intruder which has already gained a foothold. That we survive at all shows the effective counterattacking ability of our immune defense. But the time gap is where most of our terrible failures begin.

[76]

Nowhere in our life is this time gap in our defenses, the time lag between attack and defense, more critical or more obvious than in the period just after birth. Raised in the sterile world of the uterus, with no exposure to any infective agents, our children are suddenly thrust out into the polluted world, assaulted from the moment of their birth by microbes that want nothing more than to kill them, to use their hearts and lungs for their own existence.

A newborn child, never before attacked by microbes, does not have any of his own antibodies in his circulation, and his immune system would be unable to process an attacker quickly enough to get it before it gets him. The skin does hold off some, but the rest would simply flood into the infant's body through his ears and mouth, his throat and pharynx, a leaking umbilical cord, his stomach or lungs.

There would still be his granulocytes and macrophages available for defense, and they might catch some of the invaders, but most of the microbes would outflank them and get away to destroy the newborn, killing him before he had a chance to live.

And so our evolution, under the enormous pressure of keeping us always protected, has devised for each of our children an elegant legacy. We come into this teeming world with the antibodies of our mothers inside us, billions of them preformed, fully prepared to protect us as they have been protecting her. Antibodies are given the child against all the organisms that through her life the mother has been exposed to. They will cross the placenta and concentrate in the baby's body before birth. Nothing is missed since the mother's immune system is geared to fight them all—the bacteria that cause scarlet fever, whooping cough, typhus, typhoid, pneumonia, meningococcemia, the poisons that cause diphtheria and tetanus, the viruses that cause chicken pox, mumps, measles, polio or herpes.

Our mother's antibodies protect us until our immune system can begin to make our own. The first antibodies we make even as adults are always of the IgM type. Being larger than the others, they are physically the least disruptable and the most deadly to attackers. Yet it has been known for years that a day or two after infection begins—any infection—our plasma cells suddenly stop production of the more effective IgM antibodies and quite unexpectedly switch over and begin producing antibodies of the smaller, less effective IgG type.

There were many theories proposed for this changeover: that the body during evolution opted for the production of the smaller and faster IgG antibodies rather than the larger, slower IgM kind; that we are better served by a large number of the smaller type than by a small number of the large type. But now we know the reason for the switchover, why our body, to our obvious detriment, stops producing the more effective IgM antibodies, best suited for our own individual protection, and begins to produce the smaller IgG's. It was an evolutionary decision; nature, wiser than we are, decided to protect the children first, even if it means less protection for ourselves, perhaps even the sacrifice of our own lives, so that our children might have the advantage. It is all related to a simple act of physics, to the chemistry that gave rise to life and still sustains it. The IgM molecule, for all its effectiveness, is simply too big to cross the placenta.

The placenta is an evolutionary device, an organ that has evolved to allow us to keep our young within us, protected from the outside world until they are ready to survive in it. It is in reality a physical barrier, a checkpoint between mother and fetus that allows the chemical building blocks, the raw materials for fetal growth to get through. It allows the necessary oxygen, sugars, sodium and chloride, the vitamins, minerals, fats, calcium and phosphorus to cross over from the mother's circulation into her child's, while at the same time potentially dangerous materials are kept out—materials like the mother's hormones that would be destructive to embryonic growth, foreign particles like fat globules, bits of debris or even microorganisms themselves that would get in the way of fetal development and cause malformations. The smaller-size compounds and salts cross the layers of the placenta, fitting easily through the gaps in its cellular structure; the larger compounds do not. It is that simple.

For the most part the placenta is a barrier based only on the size of the material that tries to get through. The IgG antibody is just able to make it across, to get into the fetal circulation, while the IgM, being larger, must stay in the mother's circulation, along with her other proteins and enzymes. It is the ability of the IgG antibody molecule to cross the placenta that allows us to continue to exist.

Indeed, so important is the continuous presence of antibodies in the circulation of living things, so crucial for survival, that nature has arranged to make sure there is no moment of antibody lag, that antibody levels run in a continuous line from generation to generation. So significant are these levels that nature has even manipulated behavior patterns to make sure the chemistry of defense is always maintained. In animals like the pig, whose placenta is too thick to allow the passage of even the smaller IgG antibodies, the first act of the newborn piglet is to seek out the mother's nipple. With barely the energy to keep breathing, it forces itself to take one suck, just one, but it is enough. At delivery the mother's milk is supersaturated with IgG antibodies; only at that time is her milk so full of antibodies. With that one single suck, the piglet absorbs enough IgG molecules into its circulation to protect it until its own antibody defense can be brought up to normal.

You can almost picture the scenario. At one time in evolution, both IgG and IgM antibodies were produced at the same rate, but only the IgG antibodies were able to cross the newly developing placental structure simply because they were small enough to do it. At birth the newborn with these antibodies in him had a greater chance to survive than the infant with none. Whether a few molecules or a lot, the balance was tipped toward survival, and gradually the mothers whose cells produced more IgG antibodies than IgM were selected by evolution. They were the ones whose infants prospered, so the ability to make the placental-transferable IgG antibodies was one ability passed on, until today it is the IgG producers, those like ourselves, who are alive.

But the system is not perfect. It is true that right before birth our mother's IgG antibodies do accumulate in our circulation; in fact, they are pumped in to such an extent that at birth a human newborn has a higher concentration of IgG antibodies in his body than his mother has in hers, nature depleting her at the end so her own can better survive. But the transferred IgG molecules do not contain the antibodies against all the microbes we shall meet. The newborn's mother may have missed some; she may not have been attacked herself by certain microbes, so she has none of those antibodies to give him. In addition, there are microbes even today that only the bigger and stronger IgM antibodies will work against. The newborn is unprotected against such IgM-responsive organisms. But evolution has taken care of this, too.

In our mother's milk, as in all her secretions, is the third kind of antibody, the large IgA type. As soon as the infant begins to breast-feed, his mouth and throat, stomach and intestines are coated with molecules of his mother's IgA antibodies. These do not get into his body but coat his linings, and like the piglet, he is protected even from microbes which, once inside him, only the IgM antibodies would control. There is no more than an hour or two that an infant is not totally protected.

But these maternal antibodies, whether IgA or IgG, do not last long. Like any protein they soon decay; their numbers in the newborn gradually decrease. The attacks of the staph and strep, the adeno and herpes viruses will continue, but the infant has been given the time he needs to begin making his own antibodies. The two or three months that the maternal antibodies circulate within him are enough for him to build up his own supply, and from then on he is on his own.

What antibodies do in essence is very simple. Once the attacking organism gets through the outer defenses of the body, through the skin or the moist, warm mucous membranes of the nose, mouth or GI tract, once it gets into the bladder or the body proper, the antibodies that have already been made against the invader couple with the antigens on its surface and cling to the cell wall of the bacterium or virus. The antibody fits snugly onto the antigen. The antibody is incredibly small, no more than one-thousandth the size of a bacterium—but it sticks there to the antigen, like a bit of moss clinging to the bark of a tree, and that is enough. If the foreign substance is a poison, the antibody by coupling with the antigen can neutralize it, so that the toxin circulates harmlessly.

With microbes it is different; the antibodies do not actually harm the bacteria or viruses themselves. They can cause them to clump together, and because of this clumping add a little weight to the microbes and perhaps slow them down a bit, but it is like trying to slow down a freight train by putting a ball and chain on one of its wheels. They also make it easier for granulocytes to phagocytize. But what the antibodies really do is something quite new in evolution, something so startling and so deadly that it surprised the early immunologists as much as it still startles us today.

In truth, antibodies do not harm the bacteria they cling to, but once attached to the microbe's surface they unlock a series of physical events which leads to the microbe's death. Like innocent bystanders who have set in motion a catastrophe, they sit there on the microbe's surface and watch silently, apparently unconcerned, while all hell breaks loose around them.

7

Our Immune System: The Killers

SINCE THE EXPERIMENTS of the eighteen-eighties we have known that blood plasma by itself, without white cells, could kill microorganisms as well as clump them together. We knew even then how the microbes were killed, that they were literally blown apart. One second the bacteria were there in the blood-stream and the next they were shattered, broken open.

Those early researchers knew they could heat human plasma to 56 degrees Centigrade (132 degrees F.) and destroy its ability to blast apart bacteria, but not its ability to clump them. Clearly, the two functions were separate, and the real killing of bacteria had nothing to do with antibodies but with something else.

Today we know that each of us carries in his blood besides antibodies and white cells the third, and perhaps most important, part of our immune system, a group of nine separate proteins made in the liver and delivered to our circulation in such great amounts that every cubic centimeter of blood at any one time contains milligram amounts of them. The nine taken together have been given the strange name of "complement," and the nine individual proteins making up the "complement system" are called, in order, C^1, C^2, C^3, C^4, C^5, all the way up to the final component, C^9.

The name was based on an early misunderstanding of what these proteins did. The first immunologists thought they complemented the action of the antibodies. They did not realize it was the other way around, that the antibodies complemented the action of these nine proteins.

It must have taken millions of years for our body to assemble this group of nine killer serum proteins, to be able to fit them all together, all the components, so that when all were activated they would together destroy any living microorganism. Survival is the powerful force in nature. Try to destroy all the cockroaches in a kitchen, or the mold in a closet, try to get rid of the ahlwives in the Great Lakes or the mosquitoes in your park and you will see how difficult it is to kill 100 percent of anything. It is virtually an impossible task; one or two of everything will always survive. Yet that is the exact demand that we place on our body, that we have always placed on it.

Our battles against microbes have never been a war of percentages; every microbe that enters our body has to be destroyed, not 98 percent of them or 99, but 100 percent. It has to be total war; not one single enemy can be left alive. Just one survivor, by continuing to grow, would eventually mean death, and so all have to be eliminated. Our body accomplishes this truly amazing feat through its evolutionary assemblage of the nine complement proteins, which kill by taking advantage of one of the most basic facts of life, a fact so fundamental that without it there can be no life: the cellular necessity to keep the inside in and the outside out.

For life to develop, more and more chemically interrelating units had to be joined together; continually developing chemical sophistication and ever greater biological efficiency meant a more elaborate internal cellular structure, an ever increasing concentration of materials, of proteins, enzymes, hormones, DNA, RNA, microsomes, salts and minerals.

As evolution progressed, the inside of those first cells, being packed with ever greater numbers of enzyme systems, became more concentrated than the water around them. At some time

[83]

the concentration of materials inside those earliest cells must finally have become so high that the water around them began to be drawn into the cells themselves, flowing, as water always does, from a less concentrated into a more concentrated area. The cells swelled, and their newly developed internal structures began to come apart, to float away one from the other. There must have been millions of years when there was no evolution at all, when every time a new molecular system evolved within a cell, a bit more water flowed in to disrupt it. A silent time when life was at a standstill, until one cell or more than one, trying to outdistance its neighbor, developed a system within its own external membrane, a chemical pump right there in the surrounding membrane itself which could expel whatever excess water flowed in.

The evolutionary advantage of this pump was so beneficial to the cells that had it that soon they were able to increase the sophistication of their internal machinery and gradually become not only the dominant cells in those early seas, but the only cells. All life proceeded from them; all cells from then on had that pump in their outer membrane. It became an absolute necessity for existence. If it broke down or was destroyed, the water would flow in and the cell literally be drowned. There was no if or maybe about it, so those membrane pumps remained.

This early situation of increasing concentration of materials inside living cells not only remains, but today has become even more critical. Every modern cell is so sophisticated, so highly packed with internal structures that its insides are always higher in concentration than whatever fluid it is in, sea water or our body's own tissues. So great is the difference in concentration that if the membrane pump fails, or if the cell dies, the water flows in, the cell swells, and like a balloon filling with air, explodes. The same thing happens if an accident occurs, if a hole or crack opens up in the cell's surface. A hole in any cell wall means death to that cell. It was this purely physical fact, the difference in concentration between the inside of a cell and the fluids that naturally surround it, that our body in its wisdom has taken advantage of, using it to protect us.

So potent is the production of cellular holes to cellular death, so biologically devastating to all living things, that even a single crack, no matter how small, as soon as it occurs is the same as death itself. In a world of confusion and uncertainty, vagueness and probabilities, the result of that single hole is completely and utterly certain. Nature had only to develop the right tool and whoever had it would be totally armed. The proteins of the complement system are that tool; and we carry that weapon within us, ready to explode on command, to detonate when needed.

When activated, the nine complement components unite to make a microscopically small doughnut-shaped hole in any cell wall. The complement proteins assembling themselves on a bacterial cell blow it open, exploding through the microbe's protective outer covering like an armor-piercing shell. But like any explosive, the complement system is as blind as it is potent and, when ignited, will blast a hole in any cell, be it friend or foe, bacterium cell or a normal kidney cell, heart-valve or blood-vessel wall. Like any weapon, it had to be controlled to be effective. Nature had to take the additional evolutionary step of making sure it went off where it was supposed to, and this it did by the use of antibodies. Indeed, so potent is the complement system that the control had to be there before it could even begin to be assembled. The hagfish's blood can clump bacteria, it has antibodies in it, but it cannot kill bacteria; it has none of the complement proteins. The killing comes later in evolution.

The probability is that once antibodies had developed, the components of complement quickly began to evolve, each new protein of the system giving the animal an ever greater survival edge. Over hundreds of millions of years, the whole system gradually evolved; but as with the granulocytes, it was again the antibodies that were the key to its success, indeed to the complement system working at all.

It is easy to picture the havoc that could be caused if the complement proteins were activated anywhere but directly on the surface of an invader; even close to the invader some of the activated particles could miss, be carried off in the currents of circulation or simply skid off the bacterium and blast a hole in some surrounding cell or vessel, injuring normal tissues. Nature, aware of the power of its weapon, handled even that concern by making sure that the antibodies which activated the complement system were not free-floating, but only those which had already become fixed to the antigen on the microbe's surface.

[85]

We still don't know exactly how it happens, but when an antibody molecule fixes to its antigen on a microbe's surface—physically couples with the antigen—the antibody changes its shape. A special area somewhere on the antibody molecule itself is then opened up by this shape change, and the newly exposed site, opened to the circulation, activates any passing C^1, the first component of complement. Since this opening of an active site specific for complement only happens to an antibody already clinging to the surface of a microbe, the complement is activated right where it should be, right up against the one cell wall our body wants to shatter.

The sequence of the complement system's activation has recently been worked out. It is astonishing what the body does, how up to the very last moment before detonation by using all nine components it tries to minimize its chance of error. The first protein component of complement does nothing but combine with the active site of the antibody already on the surface of the microbe. With that combination it, too, changes shape. A new combining site in it opens up, and C^2, the second protein component of complement passing by in the bloodstream, fixes to that site. In a kind of fail-safe way, beginning with the activation of the first component of complement by an antibody already clinging to a bacterium, that fixation activates the second component, and so on until all nine components are assembled on the bacterial surface. None can be activated until the component directly preceding it has been activated, and with the final activation of the ninth complement protein the hole is blasted through the bacterium's outer wall. It all happens within tenths of a second, long before the bacterium can divide or even try to move away.

WITH THE UNDERSTANDING of the complement system and all that was already known about antibodies, granulocytes and macrophages, the scientists thought they had the whole picture. But even with their discovery of the complement system, there was still one great unexplained inconsistency in it all. Children born without the ability to make antibodies did not succumb right away, they lingered for at least a year or two before they died. If antibodies were so important, so crucial to all the body's immune defenses, indeed apparently necessary for every part of the immune system to work, why didn't these children die immediately? What kept them alive for that year or two?

In all the excitement with granulocytes, amid all the new discoveries about antibodies and how they work, the insights into the components of complement, those children were always there to confound the theories. Without an antibody in their system, they managed to survive at least for a while.

One man wondered. In the early nineteen-fifties, Louis Pillemer began a series of experiments which would eventually contribute to his suicide. He took human blood, and mixing it with substances he had extracted from the cell walls of yeasts, found that the complement system was activated. He called the material in the blood that combined with the yeast cell wall, and so activated the complement proteins, "properdin."

But the medical dogma at the time was that antibodies played the pivotal role in all bodily defenses. Those who had developed and supported this dogma, who had used it to rise to the heights of academic medicine, to become professors and medical administrators, would not tolerate the concept of a substance in the blood which was not an antibody but could still combine with the surface of microorganisms and activate the complement system. They attacked the researcher and his work.

When the properdin papers were presented, they were immediately challenged by those in control of medicine, academicians demanding to know of the researcher if he was sure, really sure, that antibodies were not present in his serum samples. When Pillemer answered that by all the newest means for antibody detection available he had not found any, they countered that the newest methods were just not good enough; antibody *had* to be present. His papers were refused publication.

The dogma then, as we have seen, was that antibodies, more specifically those produced against invading microbes, attached to those microbes and by that attachment either made them more susceptible to the phagocytosis of granulocytes or activated the components of complement. Pillemer's discovery of a nonimmunologic protein circulating in people's blood that activated complement did not fit the accepted pattern. "How could it?" the experts demanded. "If properdin is not an antibody, then how does it know what to attack? Why would it not attack everything?" Pillemer was shouted down as a heretic. In 1954 he committed suicide in his laboratory.

How much of his death was caused by those who would not listen and how much by his own personal problems and concerns, we'll never know. In any case, he was not the first nor will he be the last person martyred to science, beaten down for his "radical" beliefs.

As immunologic research continued, it soon became obvious that Pillemer was right; the results of experiment after experiment could only be explained by the presence of a circulating nonimmunologic substance in the blood, a substance that was not an antibody but could nevertheless combine with bacteria and activate complement. We now know that there is such a substance present in the bloodstream and that it is a protein somewhat larger than most antibodies. Apparently somehow in evolution, to fill the gap between the time when a new microbe invaded the body and the body could get around to making the right antibody and recirculate it back through the bloodstream to couple with the attacker, the body developed this nonimmunologic protein, this substance which could attach itself to any bacterium getting through the skin, no matter what the type, and which could, like its more complicated and sophisticated helper, the antibody, activate complement and blast the microbe apart long before it could move even an inch farther into the body and well before any antibody could possibly have reached it.

Properdin is now realized to be an important backup protein to our immunologic defenses. Its presence in our bloodstream is why children with immunodeficiency diseases do not die immediately. But they still die within a short time; the properdin system by itself is not enough. No one part of our defense system is ever enough. We need all of it to survive, and like any diverse and complicated system made up of many parts, in order to work properly it needs an overall controlling force, a central coordinator, something to direct the system and make sure that all its parts interact and work together.

There has to be such a central coordinator. How else could the body know time after time exactly what antibodies to make, precisely what kind to produce? How do the granulocytes always know where to go? Why do some reactions contain granulocytes and others lymphocytes? What directs it all? Where is it?

Today we know. The answer was there all along, discernible in every blood smear but ignored—the mastermind of our whole immune system.

8

Our Immune System: The Mastermind

WE HAVE ALL FELT the lymph nodes in our neck; small glands that swell up and may or may not become painful when we have a sore throat or tonsillitis. The Greeks and Romans felt them, too, and as astonishing as it may seem, until barely twenty years ago we believed what they told us about them—that these lymph glands acted as nothing more than filters, straining out the bacteria and poisons that entered our body, capturing these foreign substances before they could go farther into the body. The Greek and Roman physicians must have done autopsies on people who died from infections and found wherever they looked that the lymph glands near the infected area were always swollen and enlarged, not only the easily felt superficial nodes in infections of the skin or tonsils but those deeper down in the abdomen and chest, and down even farther in the very core of the body, around the heart and the aorta, wherever there was an infection or abscess nearby. The ancient theory of filtration and trapping of microbes held through the centuries, even when microscopic sections of those swollen nodes were finally being done and showed no microorganisms in them, not one.

Lymph nodes are distributed all over our body—in our neck and under our arms, in our legs, behind our knees and elbows, in our stomach and intestines, up and down our arteries and veins, surrounding our heart, lying between our lungs, around our liver and gall bladder—in fact everywhere, and are connected with one another by very thin-walled channels that run throughout the body alongside our arteries and veins. Actually, these lymph channels comprise the second great, if poorly understood, circulatory system of our body.

Most of what we know about these lymph glands and their connection has been discovered within the last five years. The Greeks and Romans were partially correct: our lymph glands do swell up during infections. Have a strep-throat infection, and the lymph nodes in your neck will get larger. Cut your arm, fail to take care of it, let it get infected, and the next thing you will notice will be the glands under your arm, in the armpit, swelling up. Get a boil on the back of your leg, and the lymph nodes in your groin draining that leg will become red and swollen as they double or triple in size. However, the swelling occurs not because they are filtering out infectious materials, but because the cells that make up those glands, the lymphocytes, are taking it upon themselves to divide and multiply, gearing up to make the immunologic fight that will in the end decide whether you live or die. These lymphocytes comprise the mastermind of our immune system.

The earliest microscopists dissecting parts of the body— among them Virchow, one of the greatest anatomists of all time —saw that lymph nodes, no matter from where they were taken, were filled with thousands of cells exactly like the lymphocytes he found on his blood smears circulating in the blood-stream, alongside the granulocytes. In the lymph nodes draining an infected area, Virchow would always find an increased number of these cells. Occasionally, on sections of more swollen nodes removed from infected areas, he would even find some of the lymphocytes dividing, forming more of themselves. But neither he nor anyone else made anything of this observation.

The problem then was the same problem that faced scientists up until a decade ago—losing the forest for the trees. The various parts of the immune system were discovered here and there; the granulocytes and macrophages were found to originate in the bone marrow; complement and properdin proteins were made in the liver; antibodies obviously were made by plasma cells, which seemed to be everywhere; lymphocytes were formed in the lymph nodes. But the idea that they were all connected—indeed had to be—is only a recent understanding.

Everything was too well organized, all the parts meshed too well together to be left each to its own chances. They had to be part of a complete, well-integrated system. Yet, where was it? It is easy to find the cardiovascular system: our heart, arteries and veins. Our digestive system begins at the mouth and ends at the rectum. The nervous system is made up of our brain, spinal cord and nerves. It is a rule of nature that structure precedes function: in order to digest, you need a stomach; in order to see, you need eyes. Since we obviously had an immune system, the question remained: Where was it? Not just its parts, but its entirety.

It took, as so many great achievements do, the tireless effort of one committed man to find the answer to this question. A brilliant doctor, a pediatrician who was to become a leading immunologist, Robert A. Good felt sure there must be some overall control to our immune system, and that finding it and how it worked would mean the conquering of much suffering and the elimination of most disease. He perservered and found the answer. With an amazing mind able to synthesize vast amounts of seemingly unrelated material, Good put together all that was known about immunology, and with some dazzling insights of his own came up with discoveries so simple yet so bewildering that at first they were disbelieved.

What Good discovered, and what an equally committed and brilliant woman, Ms. De Sousa, working in Glasgow, later documented, was that we do indeed have an immune system but that unlike all the other systems of the body which are in one place, or whose parts are physically connected, our immune system is too important, has too much to do, has to react too quickly for our body to have it all in any one place. So nature dispersed the system, distributing it throughout our body, putting it next to every organ, near every limb, close to every surface.

Good and De Sousa showed that the lymph nodes scattered throughout the body house our immune system, and that the system is ultimately made up of cells called lymphocytes. Those cells do it all, and it is their development and their odyssey to and from their home in the lymph nodes that is not only one of the most astonishing events in all of nature but the basis for all our immune defenses as well.

Seen on blood smears by the earliest anatomists to make use of the microscope, these cells were ignored because they just seemed to be there in the bloodstream, side by side with the granulocytes. They didn't have granules, they didn't attack bacteria, they couldn't even move under their own power; they seemed only to be carried along in the currents of the circulation. Over a hundred years ago Virchow had observed rather offhandedly that in any inflammatory process there would be a slight increase of these lymphocytes in the bloodstream, but that was all. The granulocytes ate bacteria, but the lymphocytes just sort of floated around. No one connected the increase in circulating lymphocytes with the increase in lymphocytes in the lymph nodes draining infective sites, or had any idea that this increase in numbers in both places was the beginning act in a fight which these cells had been making and getting better at for a little over a billion years.

It was only twenty-five years ago, with the development of radioactive tracer techniques, that Coleman labeled the circulating lymphocytes. When he put them back into the bloodstream and followed their course throughout the body, he was startled to find that the lymphocytes he had injected did not just bang around the body indiscriminately, drifting here and there; instead, they all followed a single, relentless, undeviating route. Seemingly without any mode of locomotion, they moved quickly through the bloodstream, out into the tissues of the body, through the heart and the muscles, the kidneys and liver, then into the closest lymph channel and back again to the nearest lymph node, then out again, back into the bloodstream and from there into the internal organs, through them, and then back again through the thin-walled lymph vessels to the nearest lymph node and then out again, in an endless cycle.

Coleman learned something else equally as surprising as the fact that lymphocytes pick their paths through the body, in a sense patrol all the areas of the body, superficial and deep, on a regular basis. What he observed was that unlike the granulocytes, many of these labeled lymphocytes did not degenerate but continued to live, and not only for a week or months but for years, making their rounds a hundred times a day, untiringly. Unlike all the other white cells, they did not die, nor were they replaced. Coleman postulated from his experiments that many of our circulating lymphocytes might live as long as we do, some certainly for as long as sixty to seventy years.

If today you went to your doctor and he took some blood from the vein in your arm, labeled your circulating lymphocytes and reinjected them into that same vein, they would travel up your arm into the superior vena cava—the large vein draining all the blood from the whole upper part of your body—and from there into your heart. Carried on the blood flow, they would tumble through the heart itself past the heart valves, and like a barrel over Niagara Falls, out into the turbulent flow of the aorta, then into the smoother flow of the medium-size arteries and from there into the small, slow-moving flow of the tissue capillaries. Once in the tissues themselves, these lymphocytes somehow leave the capillaries and move out into the organ.

They can travel past the cells of the kidneys, the liver, the muscles of your hands or fingers, the fat of your stomach or legs, and then, once through the organ, into the nearest lymph canal and back to the nearest lymph node. They move through the lymph node, past all the other lymphocytes there, and out again into the veins, for the trip back to the heart, where they move out again into the bloodstream and off to another part of the body where again they travel out into the organs and back to the nearest lymph node, touching their brother and sister lymphocytes as they pass through it, and then back once again into the veins. The tracer experiments showed that at any one moment in time we have all our circulating lymphocytes out traveling through all the various parts of our body.

If we could label all your circulating lymphocytes and then take you into an X-ray room and put you behind a fluorescent screen so that the labeled cells would show up wherever they were, you could look down at any part of your body and see them shining up at you through your skin. Every part of you would be filled with these tiny twinkling dots.

But unchanged and seemingly unchanging, what could they be doing? Why their endless, though precisely controlled trips to and from their lymph nodes? It was Good who finally understood their seemingly meaningless odyssey. From his own work, and that of countless others, he put it all together. His discovery was as brilliant as it was simple, and while it took fifteen years to definitely prove his findings, now all agree with him.

What Good found was that except for the granulocytes, our entire immune system, every part of it, as diverse as it may seem, comes from lymphocytes. The plasma cells that make our antibodies, once lymphocytes themselves, are derived from them. And the cells which transmit antigenic information to the plasma cells, telling them what kind of antibodies to make, also the cells that unlike the granulocytes attack viruses and even go after cancer cells, that bring about the rejection of transplanted organs, are all lymphocytes. Everything immunologic that happens in our body comes from these white cells with no granules, which fill all our lymph nodes and travel so persistently through the body.

Good showed that all the lymphocytes come from the few primitive cells lining the embryonic yolk sac that forms when we are just beginning to develop as embryos. During fetal growth these primitive cells move from the yolk sac in one of two directions: they migrate either to the lymph glands developing near the embryonic stomach or to a tiny gland in the neck called the thymus. Good and De Sousa proved that something happens in these places that changes those primitive pre-lymphocytic cells into what are called T or B lymphocytes—two kinds of mature lymphocytes that look exactly alike under the microscope but act totally different when coming to our defense. Those primitive pre-lymphocytic cells developing under the influence of the thymus become T lymphocytes, and those under the influence of the lymph nodes near the embryonic stomach, the B type.

After the process that effects these changes, the mature T and B cells move out from the lymph nodes near the thymus or the stomach back into the fetal circulation and finally, in some as yet unknown fashion, find their way into the embryonic and still empty lymph nodes beginning to develop all over the body, where they fill them and take up a permanent lifelong residence. The outer parts of each lymph node is filled with the B-cell lymphocytes, the inner parts with T cells. Both types sit there, one close to the other. Every so often a few lymphocytes are released into the bloodstream to circulate throughout the body. With that beginning circulation we are finally ready to make the fight that we all have to make.

And now, thanks to Good and to others, we finally know exactly how that fight is made. If you cut your hand and a bacterium enters through the skin, antibodies already formed from a previous attack or properdin couple with it. But if that bacterium has never entered the body before, one of our circulating lymphocytes will within a short time—minutes, sometimes seconds—touch it. We are not sure at all about what happens in that touching, but we know the results: one circulating lymphocyte somehow picks the antigen off the attacker's surface, and acting as messenger quickly carries the information back to the nearest lymph node draining that area. When it passes through the node it goes either to the B-cell area or the T-cell area, depending on its own inner knowledge of what exactly must be done to protect us from that particular microbe. If it touches a B cell, that cell immediately begins to change; its shape elongates and it changes into a plasma cell, virtually a protein factory that makes antibodies which fit exactly the antigen the circulating lymphocyte brought back with it. In an amplification system second to none, one messenger lymphocyte can in its passage through the lymph node literally touch thousands of separate B cells, stimulating each to form a plasma cell, all of which acting together will then go on to produce billions of specific antibodies. These, released into the bloodstream, will flood into the infected areas to go after the attacking microbes.

It is only within the last two years that we have discovered another event which can occur when a messenger lymphocyte brings back antigen information to the nearest lymph node—an event that turns on the second part of our immune response, our cellular defense.

Our antibodies, complement, properdin, granulocytes and macrophages protect us against bacteria and fungi. But our other enemies, viruses and parasites—because they are intracellular microbes, microbes that infect us by getting inside healthy cells—must be handled differently. Reacting to such infections, the messenger lymphocytes go to the T-cell area of the node rather than the B, and by touching a T cell, cause it to transform itself from a sedate cell sitting quietly in the node to what is called a killer lymphocyte which then leaves the node and move out into the circulation to attack the infected cell all by itself, without the aid of antibodies, granulocytes or complement.

It is the release of these killer T cells that accounts for the increase in circulating lymphocytes which the early microscopists noted during infections, particularly viral infections. We now know unequivocally that the killer T cells are involved in stopping viruses, controlling abnormal cancer cells and intracellular parasites, and in rejecting foreign skin grafts and transplanted organs.

Viruses are intracellular microbes. They infect us by getting inside our cells and taking over the cells' own protein machinery, making the cell produce more of them instead of the proteins or compounds it usually makes, eventually killing the cell and then moving on to infect other, nearby cells. Antibodies can be made against some viruses, sticking to their surface and keeping them from getting into our cells in the first place. But many viruses never get into the bloodstream where our antibodies and our complement, properdin and granulocytes can get at them; they infect us by getting into our body, traveling internally from tissue cell to tissue cell, never exposing themselves to our humoral defenses. Many of the viruses that cause encephalitis, hepatitis and some flu-like illneses are of this kind. It is our killer lymphocytes that must stop their spread. Indeed, it is against these intracellular enemies—viruses, parasites and rickettsial organisms—that our cellular defenses evolved.

During viral infections a circulating lymphocyte will in its rounds to and from its lymph node eventually come into contact with a viral-infected cell. Such a cell is so sick that even its surface structure is changed; the configuration of proteins making up its outer membrane becomes slightly different. The circulating lymphocyte will touch the infected cell's surface, recognize the changed part as foreign—as an antigen—and picking it off, carry it back to the nearest node, touch the T lymphocytes, transfer the information, and in the process transform the T cells into killers which will seek out the virally infected cells and couple with the antigen on their surface the same way that antibodies fix to bacteria.

Once a killer T lymphocyte couples to the surface of an infected cell, its own internal protein cell-killing machinery turns on. The coupling with the infected cell is the chemical switch that transforms the T cell into a killer cell. Chemicals are produced; compounds which evolved hundreds of millions of years ago begin to be made within the lymphocyte that diffuse out of these killer T cells like poison gas out of a canister, entering the infected cell, killing the virus, stopping the viral spread, giving our body the chance to regenerate itself.

It is these killer T cells released from our lymph nodes that we now think are involved with all types of what we have begun to call the "delayed immune responses," immune responses which have nothing to do with granulocytes or even with antibodies, and take a while to begin because they involve only our killer T cells. They are the kind of immune response typified by the slowly developing positive tuberculin skin-test reaction. The reason for the delay is that it takes the body time to get its circulating lymphocytes back to the nearest lymph node, for the messenger lymphocytes to stimulate the killer cells, and for these killer lymphocytes to get back into the circulation and carried to the infected area.

This is the way our body fights viral illnesses, the way we stop the flu and encephalitis, and holds in check the host of other intracellular parasites like the toxoplasmic organism that causes toxoplasmosis and the rickettsia of Rocky Mountain spotted fever. It is also the way our body mounts an immunologic attack against transplanted tissues with cell surfaces antigenically different from its own, using its killer T cells to go after these "foreign" transplanted cells in the same relentless, violent way it uses them to control disease by going after its own infected cells.

We still don't know how the antigenic information is transferred from the circulating messenger lymphocytes to the T or B cells of the lymph node, or how the B cells change themselves into plasma cells or the T cells into killer lymphocytes. No one can yet tell us how those killer T cells know where to go to attack the foreign invader or the infected cell, and more important, what exactly are the interactions between all parts of our immune system, humoral and cellular. What seems certain is that we need all the parts of our immune system working together—the T and B lymphocytes, the properdin, the complement system, antibodies, plasma cells, the macrophages and the granulocytes—to keep us healthy. A defect anywhere in any part leads to disease, to recurrent viral infections, pneumonia, and even cancer.

But step by step, with the increased understanding of our immune system, there has been a growing realization—at first scientifically vague and only whispered about but now accepted —that it can all go the other way, that all the magnificence of our immune system can be turned against the body and cause disease. It now appears that those early whisperers were right, that some of the most baffling and destructive diseases in all of medicine and surgery are in fact caused by our own immune system going crazy and attacking us, taking us to be the invader, the enemy.

The immune system, always the counterattacker, given absolutely no margin for error and always on the alert, has to make instantaneous judgments and responses. But sometimes, because it cannot afford to be wrong, it leaps too soon; sometimes it misreads the signs and launches itself at our own cells just as relentlessly as it would any foreign invader.

It took a long time to realize this could happen, and an even longer time to prove it.

9

Rh Incompatibility: The Riddle

DISEASES do not occur only after we are born. They can begin even before birth—congenital malformations, defects in organs as they are being formed: a heart that doesn't fold properly, leaving holes between its chambers; an arm that doesn't bud; a kidney that becomes a cyst; a developing brain filling with nothing but fluid. Infections, too, can destroy a child before he is born: the spirochete that causes congenital syphilis; the parasite of toxoplasmosis; the viruses of cytomegalic inclusion disease and German measles—all can cross the placenta and infect a developing child, destroying his eyes, his heart valves, his joints and bones, his muscles, brain, his kidneys and liver, before they are put to use. The miracle is not that we are born whole but that we manage to get born at all.

But the most common disease that occurs in newborns is not caused by a congenital defect or by bacteria or a virus but by the baby's own mother, by her immune system going astray and attacking the infant, in some cases resulting in her child's death even as he is being born, in other cases resulting in severe illness and lifelong disabilities. The disease is called erythroblastosis fetalis, or more commonly, Rh incompatibility. Occurring once in every 200 pregnancies, it is caused by the mother's antibodies entering her child's body and destroying the fetus' red blood cells even as they are being formed, even as they are being pumped through the infant's circulation. Hunted down by the maternal antibodies, these fetal red blood cells are destroyed wherever they are found—in the baby's capillaries and veins, in his heart or lungs. They are consumed, blasted apart by the mother's own immune system which, if not gone mad, has at least gone blind.

Not all the affected infants are born dead. Some, having only a few of their red cells destroyed, are born bloated and in heart failure, but alive. Others are born convulsing and will be mentally retarded for life. Still others become severely jaundiced. For some afflicted families, there will never be a healthy child born, each pregnancy ending in either death or disease.

Even before the beginning of recorded time, there must have been these mothers, left forever barren—their babies, one after the other, born dead or jaundiced, and the deaths explained away as being due to a scourge, to punishment, to bad thoughts, the evil eye or a diseased womb. Hippocrates and Galen, Paracelsus and Jenner—generation after generation of physicians were witnesses to this tragic phenomenon.

It was only in 1957 that a medical researcher first described a method for staining babies' red cells so that their presence could be detected even in small numbers in a mother's circulation. The method would have been no more than a trifling scientific tool if the mothers whose children were born afflicted with the Rh disease were not found to always have a few of their own diseased infants' red cells circulating in their own bloodstream. In every case, these fetal cells in the mother's circulation were all Rh-positive, whereas the mother's red cells were always Rh-negative.

Today most laymen know about the different blood groups. In the U.S. Army, for instance, every soldier has A, AB, B or O stamped on his dog tags. It is not a foolish bureaucratic concern. In 1934 Landsteiner, mixing the serum from the blood of people working in his medical laboratory with the red blood cells of others in his lab, proved for the first time that the blood of some people will clump the red cells of others, and that the red blood cells in everyone's circulation fall into one of four different but well-defined types that are as genetically determined for each of us as are our blue eyes or black hair. Landsteiner originally named these four groups with Roman numerals, I, II, III and IV; later the groups became known as type A, B, AB and O.

Landsteiner's was a simple experiment: the mixing of one person's serum with another person's red blood cells. Blood is made up of serum and red cells. The addition on a glass slide of a drop of serum from a patient with type O red blood cells in his circulation will cause the red cells of a patient with type B or AB to clump together. Landsteiner did not know why this occurred, but it was obvious to immunologists that the clumping together of the one type of red blood cells by another person's serum was similar to the ability of immunized human serum to clump together bacteria. The experiment indicated the presence in everyone's circulation of antibodies against the red blood cells of others with different blood types.

But red cells were hardly to be considered the same as foreign invading microbes. It took years to prove and more years to understand that immunologicaly there is no difference between the two. Landsteiner's work marked the beginning of our understanding not only of Rh incompatibility but of blood transfusions as well.

FROM ANCIENT TIMES men had watched their brothers bleed to death. Cauterization with red-hot pokers to close torn arteries, tourniquets, even amputation were used at one time to stop blood loss. Brutal as these methods were, they were the only way known to avoid the death that would surely follow from continued loss of blood. Time and again physicians repeating the efforts of the past tried to transfuse blood from humans. The results were almost always the same. Those who had been given the blood soon became delirious, their sudden fever burned the hands of those who held them down, and instead of bleeding to death, they died shortly of convulsions, infections, renal failure and shock. Refinements were tried. With a beginning understanding of infectious disease, physicians thought all the complications were due to bacterial contamination of the transfused blood. To eliminate this possibility they ran blood directly from the vein of one person into the vein of the patient. But chills still racked the bleeding man; delirium again gave way to convulsions, fever to death.

Even if for some reason the bleeding stopped, and the transfused person was no longer in danger of bleeding to death, he would almost surely die anyway from the transfusion. So uniformly disastrous were the results of any kind of transfusion that with blood all around—no more than an arm-vein away—bleeding to death either on the battlefield or in the operating room was held preferable to trying to give the patient blood.

With his discovery of different blood groups, Landsteiner showed why transfusions were so uniformly disastrous: each person's blood contains antibodies against another's red blood cells if those red cells are of a different type than his own. But why are the antibodies there? The people in Landsteiner's laboratory had never had transfusions, nor had they ever been attacked by someone else's red cells. Where had those antibodies present in all of us come from and why?

The answer is strictly chemical, the reason for those antibodies solely molecular. It has nothing to do with reason or sense, but rather with blindness and struggle, a continuation of the chemical warfare that began in the primeval seas and is still carried on within us today. The immune system has no recognition of our human concerns. It follows its own ways, as it always has, going after any chemical surface it reads as different, attacking the antigen, the foreign group of proteins on that surface. It does not matter what that surface is—bacteria, fungi, chemical poison, transplanted organs or red cells; as long as it is read by the circulating lymphocytes as foreign, it will be attacked. Our immune system will respond to a staphylococcus or a rabies-infected brain cell with the same tenacity and violence that it goes after a newly transplanted "foreign" kidney or a red cell of a different type.

The cell surface of every living thing is made up of proteins. If these proteins are read as foreign, any creature, any material, any particle that has these proteins on its surface—living or nonliving, organic or inorganic—will be attacked. And that is why one's blood will clump together red cells from a person with a different blood group, and that is exactly what happens when mismatched blood, blood of a different type with antigens on its surfaces that are different from the patient's own red cells, is transfused.

The antibodies we each have naturally against others' blood groups, even though we have never been exposed to them, are antibodies we have made against antigens similar to those on red cells different from our own. Some bacteria have antigens similar to the markings on red cells. So do some of the foods we eat. Whatever the cause, the antibodies are there in our circulation, so that when the mismatched blood is given, these antibodies couple immediately with the antigens on the transfused foreign red cells' surface. At the same time more antibodies are produced, complement is activated, holes are punched in the red-cell membranes, until like bacteria under attack they swell and burst apart. If the number of foreign red cells transfused is great, the reaction going on in the body of the patient is astounding—fever, sweating, delirium. The destruction can be so monumental (billions of the transfused cells being destroyed at once) that their fragments can clog all the small arteries of the patient's body, plugging them up so that the organs they serve —heart, kidneys, liver and brain—deprived of their blood supply, decay and die—eventually, if the reaction is severe enough, causing the death of the patient.

Landsteiner found only four different antigens, representing the four different blood-group antigens, on the surface of human red cells. Assured by these discoveries, bursting with new-found knowledge and buoyed by yet another victory of medical science, physicians using Landsteiner's groupings confidently began matching people's blood types and transfusing compatible blood. In 1938 two other antigens, named M and P, were also found on human red cells, but unlike Landsteiner's A, B, AB and O antigens, the M and P did not cause problems if injected into people whose own red blood cells did not have these proteins on their surface. Transfusions were given even more confidently.

But if science is exact, it can also be deadly narrow. In 1939 the physicians' confidence was suddenly and rudely shattered. In that year a woman was given what was supposedly a well-matched blood transfusion. Within minutes she suffered a near-fatal reaction. She survived, just barely.

Her doctors, confused, rechecked her own blood type

against the remaining, as yet untransfused blood. They were the same. She was A. The transfused blood was A. Even the minor groups were the same—both M—and the transfused blood was sterile, yet she had suffered a severe and almost fatal transfusion reaction. It was as if the blood she was given did not match her own, even though the lab had verified that it did. The mechanics were all appropriate; everything had been done right, yet the patient had almost died.

Her doctors then made an equally disturbing discovery. She was type A, but after the almost fatal reaction, her own blood serum now clumped red cells of every type, even types like her own; she was making antibodies against every blood group known. What had occurred with the transfusion that had not only almost killed the woman but had caused something to happen to her own bloodstream, so that now she had circulating antibodies to all blood types? She became the center of one of the greatest medical searches of modern times. All blood transfusions hung in the balance. How could transfusions, so lifesaving a procedure, be continued if suddenly, for no reason, there might be a life-threatening reaction? The reason had to be found.

Meticulously going over her history, her physicians discovered that a month before her near-fatal transfusion, this same woman had given birth to a dead fetus. A few weeks later, another woman in another part of the country, again given a supposedly well-matched blood transfusion, had a transfusion reaction and died. She, too, had recently given birth to a dead baby. The relationship between the dead newborns and these patients' own severe transfusion reactions would not be understood for over a year.

In a series of unrelated experiments being done at the time, the blood from a rhesus monkey was injected into rabbits. As was expected, the rabbits' immune system responded to the injection of the foreign red blood cells as to any foreign invader. Antibodies were produced against the rhesus monkey's red blood cells and began to circulate through the rabbits' bloodstream. When the rabbits were bled it was found, again as expected, that their blood contained antibodies against the rhesus monkey's red cells and would, if mixed on a slide with the red cells from any rhesus monkey, cause them to clump together.

[105]

What wasn't expected was that the blood from these rabbits, immunized with the red cells of the rhesus monkey, would also clump red cells from humans. Not just some humans, but like the serum of the woman who had the transfusion reactions and had survived, all human red blood cells, whatever their type.

The rabbits' blood acted the same way as the blood of the woman who had almost died. Exposed only to the red blood cells of the rhesus monkey, the rabbits had made antibodies specifically against those injected red cells. Yet those same antibodies attacked and coupled with human red cells—all, not just certain types, but all—even though the rabbits' immune system had never been exposed to one single human red-cell antigen. Since immunologists had proved that each antibody is specific for only one antigen, the only explanation was that there were markers on the surface of human red cells exactly the same as those on the rhesus monkey's red cells, and that the antibodies produced by the rabbits could not distinguish between the two; they went after human red cells as diligently and ruthlessly as they went after the monkey's.

There was no other explanation, and it made sense evolutionarily. We share a common heritage with the monkeys. Why not a common red-cell antigen? Somehow Landsteiner and the people who had discovered the M and P antigens had missed this one. Since this new red-cell antigen had been discovered by using blood from rabbits injected with rhesus-monkey red blood cells, it was called the Rh antigen.

The importance of all this is simply that human red cells contain not only blood-group antigens A, B, AB and O, M and P on their surface but also another, heretofore unknown antigen, "Rh." If red blood cells with the Rh antigen on their surface (Rh-positive cells) were injected into people with Rh-negative cells in their circulation, the potential for disaster was present.

The researchers had finally found a possible clue as to why one woman had almost died and the second had died from supposedly well-matched transfusions. The woman who was alive was checked; her own red blood cells were Rh-negative, yet her blood contained Rh-positive antibodies against the Rh antigen. She had plainly been given mismatched blood. It was nobody's fault, no one knew any better; they had typed the bloods against every antigen they thought was present, but had missed one.

To protect against further transfusion reactions, physicians began testing blood for the Rh antigen and found to their surprise that many people who were Rh-negative had by mistake been given the Rh-positive blood transfusion and that the patients, despite being given the "wrong" blood, had still done well.

That was, almost all of them. In going over a nationwide survey of records, the researchers found that in all cases of an unexplained severe reaction following one transfusion, the patient was a woman who either had recently delivered a child or had given birth to a stillborn, and these women were all found to be Rh-negative. Their husbands, though, were found to be Rh-positive, having Rh-positive cells in their circulation, and the infants' blood type, determined from umbilical-cord blood saved from these women's dead fetuses, were all found to contain Rh-positive red cells, like their fathers'.

THE RIDDLE was beginning to unfold and its implications were socially terrifying. Eighty-five percent of the white population were found to have Rh-positive cells in their circulation, 15 percent Rh-negative. Antibodies against Rh-positive cells will be produced in any Rh-negative person, man or woman, who is given a transfusion of Rh-positive cells. His or her immune system reads the Rh cells as foreign, and an immune response is mounted. Antibodies, complement, properdin, white cells, granulocytes, lymphocytes, all are mobilized, as if the person were being attacked by a microbe. The foreign Rh-positive red cells are destroyed. If the transfusion is large and a great many red cells are destroyed, a severe reaction occurs and possibly death.

But the researchers noticed that in transfused Rh-negative men, the reaction occurred only after a second transfusion with the mismatched Rh-positive cells. Obviously the first transfusion did not cause a reaction; only the second did.

The theory was proposed that the first injection of Rh-positive cells caused the production of small amounts of antibody, that this production of anti-Rh antibodies took time to occur, and since the injected cells were gone in a few days, before antibody production really got going, no reaction occurred. With the second transfusion, though, things were different; the anti-Rh antibodies were already there and destroyed the newly transfused cells, as they were being injected. The second transfusion caused a severe reaction. But those two original women and all the others suffering transfusion reactions because of Rh incompatibility had not previously had a transfusion; all they had done was give birth to stillborns. Was there a connection between the two, between these stillborns and that first sensitizing blood transfusion with mismatched Rh-positive blood cells?

It was found that there was. It begins in any Rh-negative woman when she marries an Rh-positive man. The genetics are such that the majority of children from this union will be Rh-positive. We know now, from the staining technique for fetal red blood cells, that at delivery, with the bleeding into the uterus that normally occurs, some of the baby's Rh-positive red blood cells leak across the placenta and get into the mother's circulation. This means that if it is a first pregnancy and the mother has never had a transfusion, her immune system is exposed to the Rh-positive cells of her baby for the first time only at delivery. Since it takes a few days for her own immune system to make antibodies against any foreign antigen, by the time her new anti-Rh antibodies are in her circulation hunting down any Rh-positive cells still in her body, her child is already safely free of her, on his own outside her womb, away from her blood supply and these newly circulating antibodies. The number of Rh-positive cells that usually leak across at delivery are small, so that there is no observable reaction, no injury to the mother as the Rh-positive cells are destroyed, blasted apart by her circulating antibodies and complement.

But the mother's immune system, always alert, is now primed. If she is then transfused with Rh-positive cells, she will have a severe reaction. But that is only part of it. With her next pregnancy of an Rh-positive baby, and the leakage during the pregnancy of even a few Rh-positive cells into her circulation, her antibody response will be increased ten thousand fold. This time it is her baby, too, who will be attacked. The Rh-positive antibodies are IgG's, and like any IgG antibody, will cross the border between mother and child, flow across the placenta and invade the infant's own bloodstream. Like crazed battalions suddenly let free, they begin to murder and plunder in this foreign land, destroying every Rh-positive red cell they find there. The result is, at best, anemia in the child; if the anemia is severe enough—and in many cases it will be—permanent brain damage, heart failure and stillborn deliveries are produced.

If the mother becomes pregnant a third time by the same Rh-positive husband, she will produce still more antibodies, which will cross the placenta and attack and kill her third child. With each successive pregnancy, new fetal Rh-positive cells cross into her circulation, her immune system grows stronger, more and more antibodies are formed, more cross the placenta, and each new child is attacked even more viciously than the last.

FROM 1940 ON, with an understanding of what caused Rh disease, there were only three choices: Rh-negative women were told not to marry Rh-positive men, or if already married, were counseled never to have children, or they were told to try to have only one child, hoping the mother would not be sensitized too early in the pregnancy and so go on to produce antibodies that would destroy her child before it was born.

By the late forties every pediatrician knew that the cause of these Rh infants' deaths, or of their being born diseased, was the anemia resulting from their red cells being destroyed. Those who died before they were born were suffocated by a lack of oxygen-carrying red cells. Those who lived came into the world with generalized edema, pleural effusions, pulmonary edema, large livers. Many were so anemic that they were born already in severe heart failure with heart rates of up to two hundred beats per minute; all, whatever the severity of their disease, had trouble breathing, almost all would eventually become severely jaundiced.

Such children were described by Greek physicians at least as far back as 400 B.C., but up until thirty years ago nothing could be done; the children either were born dead or lived to be damaged or retarded. It was only when the immunologic cause of the children's problem was discovered—when it was realized that the disease was not infectious or congenital but the result of the children's own red blood cells being destroyed by their mothers' antibodies, and that all their symptoms were due to their coming into the world anemic with their red cells gone —that a treatment became possible. If the cause of these children's disease was anemia, why not give them Rh-negative blood to replace what they had lost? And so the idea of doing exchange blood transfusions on diseased Rh-incompatible children was proposed. By the early forties there was enough technology to make such transfusions possible. Tiny catheters were developed that could be placed into a newborn's umbilical vein, blood preservation had reached the point where blood could safely be used even after being stored for days, and monitoring equipment was available to check the children during the exchange.

The first exchange transfusion on a severely ill child was done in the mid-forties. A newborn, in heart failure, bloated to twice his normal size, was rolled in his incubator to the pediatric intensive-care unit, where under the surgical lights his abdomen was cleaned and a catheter was placed into his umbilical vein and threaded up that vein until it reached the large vein carrying blood directly back to his heart. Syringes and valves were connected to the catheter. The poor thin watery blood, almost totally empty of red blood cells, was exchanged for normal Rh-negative blood collected from Rh-negative donors. The objective of the exchange transfusion was the removal of the baby's anemic blood and its replacement with blood containing normal amounts of red blood cells which the Rh-positive antibodies in his circulation would not attack.

There were many things that could go wrong in the exchange transfusion which did and still do. It was not only a matter of technique, of being able to place the catheter without tearing the umbilical vein and causing a hemorrhage, or pushing it up too near the tiny heart and causing a deadly cardiac arrhythmia. There was also the problem of how fast the blood was to be put in, or how fast it was removed. And the problem of infection. One third of all the blood used in exchanges contains the hepatitis virus, while refrigerated blood itself, even if still sterile, breaks down and turns severely acidic. Finally, there was the risk that the catheters could cause thrombosis, tissue damage and even death. All this, in addition to working over a human being weighing no more than four or five pounds, made the procedure fairly risky.

Exchange transfusions for infants afflicted with Rh incompatibility disease is still a life-threatening procedure; the risks, even with the new refinements of cardiac monitoring, newer catheters, continuous arterial sampling of blood acidity and electrolytes, of calcium and potassium levels, better blood storage, the use of antibiotics, are still substantial. Seventy percent of these ill infants are salvaged by the exchange procedure, but not all of these emerge free of brain damage. Enthusiasm for exchange transfusion, even initially, has never matched the hopes of those early pediatricians who realized that all the problems in these Rh-diseased children were caused by their anemias and could theoretically be treated by correcting their anemias with transfusions. The exchanges just didn't work that well and pediatricians still had to tell prospective Rh-positive fathers and Rh-negative mothers what to expect—a good chance that if they had any children, they would be born dead or severely damaged.

But there was one hope: one fact didn't make sense.

10

The Riddle Solved

FROM THE GENETICS INVOLVED, researchers were able to calculate the expected incidence of Rh disease. What they found was that the actual number of newborns affected was much lower than anticipated. Why was this? Why were some children spared who should, according to the figures, have been ill or been born dead? All efforts began to center on finding the answer to this why.

It was the clinical medical researchers—starting with the confusing mathematics of the disease and pursuing from there one lead into the next, and the basic medical scientists chemically defining each of their new discoveries—who finally together found the answer, and with it the way not merely to treat the disease but to prevent it. Neither kind of researcher could have done it alone, and their combined efforts demonstrate the best of modern medicine.

THE CLINICAL RESEARCHERS and the basic medical scientists say they both do the same thing, but there is a difference: the basic medical scientist has no clinical responsibilities. Like a nuclear physicist concerned with quantum numbers and degrees of strangeness, he deals with problems, not with people.

Just how exactly does the hemoglobin in red cells chemically bind oxygen? How many amino cells are there in insulin? What does the cytoplasm of cells do? How exactly do chromosomes work?

Even if they have an M.D. degree, basic scientists are scientists first and doctors second, if at all. Indeed, many earn their M.D. degrees as insurance against the lean days of government support. It is easier to get grants, to pursue research interests as an M.D. than as a Ph.D., a doctor rather than merely a bright chemist or a good physiologist. A physician is more likely to be listened to and respected than a professor of biology.

These physicians are the men of medicine who today carry on the scientific tradition of the great eighteenth- and nineteenth-century chemists and physicists, believing now, as their predecessors did before them, that if you can't measure it, you don't know it; if you can't accurately describe it, you risk speaking nonsense; if your data are not reproducible, they are meaningless; that if the material you are experimenting on isn't pure, you can't work with it. Precise, analytical, these men and women are the backbone of modern medicine. By scrupulously using scientific methods to deal with test-tube systems, they are able to control all the factors in their experiments except the one they are testing for, and because of this control, are able to give definitive, quantative answers to the problems they deal with. How exactly is complement consumed? What is the precise sequence of its activation? How and where does it bind to the cell membrane? What are receptor sites on an antibody molecule? What exactly is the molecular configuration of properdin? What makes granulocytes move? How do the circulating lymphocytes pass on the antigenic information to the T and B cells?

Enders, for instance, a Nobel prize-winner, working in his lab at Harvard during the forties and fifties, was engaged in basic research. Trying to grow viruses in a test tube, he spent years figuring out the exact nutrients they needed, the oxygen saturations necessary for their growth, which antibiotics had to be added to the broths, the best tissues in which to grow them, what temperatures would be optimum. It was work with no immediate application, a supposedly very narrow part of science: defining the requirements for artificial viral growth.

Yet Enders' experiments led directly to the polio vaccine, just as the work in the early twentieth century on the nutritional requirements of the white rat had led directly to an understanding of human nutritional needs. The basic medical researchers are the pure scientists of medicine; in their definitively exact world there are either twenty-one amino acids in the alpha chain of a molecule of insulin or there are not. For them everything is out in the open; you stand or fall on the exactness, precision, rigorousness and reproducibility of your work. Indeed, it is the demand of basic research that your work should be challenged. If it cannot meet the challenge, it goes down and the researcher with it.

The basic scientists are the physicians you will probably never see. They will not come to your bedside; they will not walk down the wards or be in the nurses' area checking charts. You might see them in their white lab coats in the corridors of the hospital or medical school, or perhaps on television talking about a new discovery, or accepting a Lasker award or Nobel prize. If you want to see them, you must go to the hospital's research area, to their labs, where you will find them working late into the night to solve those problems whose answers we'll need tomorrow.

The clinical researchers, on the other hand, take their clues from their patients. They are the doctors on the wards and clinics, the physicians and professors you see on rounds, those who visit you in your room, who move through the corridors surrounded by an entourage of interns, residents and medical students. The patient is their problem, the disease and the suffering their enigma. They deal with the whole of medicine and their concerns in fact are nothing more than correlations. They carry on the traditions of Jenner and Semmelweis; they look and wonder. Jenner saw that cowpox protected people from smallpox, Semmelweis that hand-washing stopped puerperal fever. Today men like them still wonder in the same way. Since salt seems important in causing hypertension, will decreased salt intake lower high blood pressure? Is exercise important in cutting down heart attacks? Does smoking cause lung cancer? Is a simple mastectomy the best operation for breast cancer, or a radical mastectomy? What is the appropriate dose of aspirin to cut down the pain of rheumatoid arthritis? Will aspirin work on other types of arthritis?

The whole patient is there in front of the clinical researcher, and while he might intellectually be interested in exactly how aspirin works to cut down the pain in arthritis, which of the bodily systems it affects, what membranes it stabilizes, what enzyme systems it might block to reduce the fever and the joint-swelling, he does not have the time nor the mathematical background nor perhaps the laboratory interest to pursue those final biological answers. He leaves the unraveling of those mysteries to the basic scientist. His concern is people; he observes that in some diseases aspirin relieves symptoms while in others it doesn't, and then determines what dose is best for the patient without causing complications from the drug itself —bloody diarrhea and ringing in the ears.

Dealing with patients, their suffering and pain, their anxieties and fears, the joints that won't stop swelling, the scaling skin that won't heal, brain tumors that lead to vomiting, the blindness of retinal degeneration, the seizures of epilepsy, the clinical researcher's concern becomes a correlation between what is happening to the patient and what is happening in the patient's body. He cannot control all the factors, as the basic scientist can, so speculation becomes much more a part of this type of research than of basic science. Clinical-research papers cannot be as vigorously attacked or challenged as can basic-science publications, because they are not as rigorously written or controlled.

It is the difficulty in proving or disproving clinical assertions that bothers the basic scientists. Does aspirin itself really lower fever or is it the aspirin working through some other compound in the body that lowers the temperature? How can we be sure, and until we are, should aspirin be used as widely as it is? Is it really bright lights that lower bilirubin levels in jaundiced infants, or something else? Until we know, should jaundiced infants be put under those lights? What happens if the decrease in jaundice leads to a more severe problem; after all, where is the jaundice going? Do new drugs make people feel better or is it simply wanting to help the researcher succeed that makes the patient say the drug does help? Should these drugs then be released? What about side effects?

At present, research is in vogue, especially of the clinical type. Indeed, it is the new tyranny of medicine. It has become so great, so pervasive that virtually every staff man, every professor, every full-time academic appointee in every medical school, in every department of medicine, pediatrics and surgery participates in it; he virtually has to call himself "a researcher." Promotions and career depend on his research activities whatever they may be, and so they are pursued. "He's doing research" has taken on the same general notion and popular license in this age as "God's will" did in the twelfth and thirteenth centuries. But medical research pursued only in this way, science used only for self-interest and personal advancement, can and does corrupt the whole process as well as the word itself.

The Tuskegee study is a part of this type of "research" corruption: men with syphilis were left untreated to determine the natural course of the disease. They were left to die from syphilis by physicians not of the fourteenth century, but of the twentieth, "researchers" who withheld treatment and wrote their papers not under the guise of Aristotelian logic, but under the excuse of research. It is the same corruption that allowed dermatologists in the nineteen-sixties to test a new drug on medical students suffering from psoriasis, with no concern that the material in which the drug was dissolved might itself cause liver disease. There are physicians today who say they are doing research, yet flee from critical attack, and continue to write sloppy treatment protocols and try medicines when they know that the real answer might be nothing more than a change in diet or better nutrition. The grants must be gathered, the papers must be published, prestige among colleagues must continue, positions must be maintained.

As patients we are forced to pay the price for such self-service. In areas where patients, because of insurance regulations, are required to get a second medical opinion, operations are reduced from 20 to 60 percent in comparison with areas where no second opinions are asked for. In the United States, nitrates known to cause cancer in animals are allowed to be added to over 12 billion pounds of meat a year in amounts far in excess of even governmental standards. It is known beyond question that cigarette smoking causes lung cancer. Yet clinical researchers look the other way and continue to pursue their own personal interests. As a result we have the development of additional surgical procedures rather than surgical responsibility, treatments for cancer rather than prevention. It is this sort of thing that drives the basic researchers crazy and leads them to speak poorly of clinical researchers and clinical research. But as always, there are those who feel the responsibility of their patients' trust, who realize the limitations of the clinical art and are concerned first and foremost with truth and integrity. It is physicians like these—the professionals, not the careerists— who give medicine its worth, and clinical research its value. These are the ones who for ten years diligently pursued Rh disease of the newborn and finally, because they would not compromise for less, found the answers and then the cure.

THEY BEGAN their study with that simple mathematical observation: the actual incidence of Rh disease of newborns was much less than what theoretically it should have been. If one assumed random mating of the population, an Rh-negative woman had an 85 percent chance of marrying an Rh-positive man, which gave the woman, because of the genetics involved, a 50 percent chance of producing an Rh-positive fetus. Eliminating first pregnancies, in which the mothers had not yet been sensitized, and women who might have received Rh-positive blood during a pre-pregnancy transfusion, there should have been at least 50,000 Rh-disease babies born a year. On strictly scientific grounds, using the most rigidly accurate methodologies available, that's what should have happened. But the actual incidence was closer to one-tenth that number.

This one mathematical fact was available to every physician and scientist who claimed an interest in Rh disease and presumably wanted to do something about it. Yet there were only a few who saw the importance of the fact and asked the simple question "Why?"—not yet "How?" but simply "Why?" These physicians looked at the data, went over them again and came up with the only two possible answers for the discrepancy: either the red cells of the Rh-positive fetuses had not entered most of those at-risk Rh-negative mothers' circulation during the pregnancy or the delivery, or if they had entered, they had not triggered the mothers' immune response. It was one of the two. But which?

In the late nineteen-fifties researchers began trying to find out. Hundreds of old records had to be examined, compared, evaluated; the sick versus the nonsick, those afflicted with Rh versus the healthy. Meanwhile the disease went on. Was there a difference between those infants affected and those not, something that had been missed? New Rh-negative mothers being admitted to the hospital to deliver were evaluated, lab values studied, new histories and physicals taken. "What drugs have you been on? Have you had any fevers? Any children afflicted with Rh disease? Any of your children born with anemia? Have you had any miscarriages? Have you had any stillborns? Anybody in your family, any relatives you know of who have had miscarriages or given birth to stillborns?"

Everything and anything had to be considered. Some of the Rh-negative women who should have been afflicted were spared and had normal pregnancies, while others just like them in every way gave birth to diseased infants. Even as the doctors struggled to get a glimpse of where to go to find the answer, afflicted children continued to be born dead, others continued to be wasted, more became retarded, while some mysteriously were saved.

But the basic scientist had given these clinicians powerful new tools to work with. By the late fifties they could readily check for the presence of antibodies—any antibody in a person's bloodstream—and by using the fetal-red-cell staining technique could prove or disprove the presence of a baby's red blood cells in his mother's circulation. Reviewing the old records did not prove very useful; all that work did was to reaffirm the researchers' conviction that indeed infants who should have been afflicted simply were not.

It was in the new patients being admitted to the hospital that the researchers found what they were seeking. As part of their search they drew blood from Rh-negative mothers before and after delivery and found that fully 25 percent of these women had their infants' Rh-positive blood entering their own circulation right after delivery. It was easy to see why. The mixing of the child's blood with the mother's as the placenta pulled free permitted the red cells from the child, whatever his type—A, B, AB, O, M, P, Rh-positive or Rh-negative—to enter the mother's bloodstream. The time of delivery was proved for the vast majority of Rh-negative mothers to be the time of their sensitization to the Rh-positive antigen.

Red blood cells begin to appear in a developing fetus at the fourth week of gestation. By the tenth week of development they number 1,500,000 per cubic centimeter of fetal blood; in the twenty-fourth week, 3,000,000. As pregnancy proceeds, the red blood cells comprise a steadily increasing population of the fetus' developing blood volume. If these red blood cells, from the time they were first being formed, had continually leaked into the mother's bloodstream, her immune system would have had the time to manufacture Rh antibodies in sufficient amounts to cross back over the placenta and destroy her baby's red cells well before the baby was delivered, killing him before he was born. The first pregnancies were usually not afflicted, because the baby's red cells did not cross the placenta until the bleeding of delivery; until that time the mother did not have any fetal red cells in her circulation, so she did not make any Rh antibodies against them. This explained why first children were spared, but not the rest.

The physicians continued drawing bloods, watching new mothers and new children, checking the results. They knew why the first infant was spared, so they had part of the answer to why the incidence of Rh disease was less than expected. But only part. Even with the first-borns being spared, the actual incidence was still much less than expected. They knew now where the sensitization to the Rh-positive antigen occurred, and how. They had also determined that approximately 25 percent of the Rh-negative mothers had Rh-positive cells in their circulation after delivery. Yet despite this proven fact, it was soon discovered, to the doctors' disbelief, that almost one fourth of the mothers who had the Rh-positive cells in their circulation immediately after delivery did not make Rh antibodies. More important, when a short time after their delivery their blood was again checked, the Rh-positive fetal cells were gone; they had mysteriously disappeared. Not one could be found anywhere in the circulation of these mothers.

It was an astonishing discovery. Research had proved that

most, if not all, sensitizations occurred at delivery, and that if Rh-positive cells got into an Rh-negative mother's circulation, she would make antibodies that would affect subsequent pregnancies. And now it was found that a fourth of the women who should have been making antibodies, and who did indeed have Rh-positive cells in their circulation after delivery, not only did not make any antibodies at all, but had the Rh cells disappear.

The doctors drew blood sample after blood sample, arterial blood and veinous blood, but they could not find these Rh-positive cells. Perhaps it was the methods they were using; perhaps something had happened to the chemical reagents used in the tests. They rechecked their work, checked new patients, made more smears, did more tests, but the same thing continued to happen: approximately 25 percent of the mothers examined who had Rh positive cells in their circulation at the time of delivery did not have the cells there two weeks after their Rh-positive children were born. The Rh positive cells were gone, all trace of them lost.

The doctors began to look more closely at these mothers and reaffirmed their findings. In addition, it was proved that those mothers in whom the Rh-positive cells had vanished never made one Rh-positive antibody. Even with the Rh-positive cells once in their bodies, no antibodies were produced. It was as if they had never given birth to an Rh-positive baby, as if they had never been pregnant with a baby of an incompatible blood type, as if they had never had a single Rh-positive red cell in their bloodstream. On the other hand, those women who continued to have Rh-positive cells in their circulation did make antibodies and did have the children of their subsequent pregnancies diseased. The doctors checked their mathematics again. If they subtracted the number of women who should have made antibodies but didn't from the expected rates of delivery, they came close to what was actually happening.

The reason for the discrepancy between the expected number of Rh-afflicted infants and the actual, much smaller number of delivered Rh babies had been found. The discovery led eventually to the cure of the disease, just as surely as Jenner's observation that milkmaids afflicted with cowpox were spared the ravages of smallpox led to the cure of that scourge.

There was plainly something special about the mothers

who got rid of the Rh-positive cells that had entered their bloodstream. The researchers started all over again. They reviewed these mothers' charts, looked at the lab values again and again, searched for anything all these women had in common that would fit with the other single fact they had in common—that Rh-positive red cells entering their circulations had disappeared.

These researchers were working at the philosophical underpinning of science. They were involved in what science does best, searching for the common factor or factors in an observed phenomenon. They succeeded in finding it. But it took them a while, because the common factor they were searching for was not only in the mothers but in their children, too.

The answer lay not in the Rh factor, but in the other major blood groups. The doctors found that all the mothers who had had the Rh-positive cells disappear from their circulation were those who had different major blood groups than their babies. Not only were these mothers Rh-negative while their infants were Rh-positive, but they were O when their child was A, or A when he was B, or B when he was A, or O when he was AB. The Rh-positive cells had not disappeared or vanished from the mother's circulation, but being of a different major blood type than her own, they had been destroyed by the anti-A, anti-B, or anti-AB antibodies she already had in her circulation. The reason why these mothers had been spared lay in nature attacking itself, in immunology fighting immunology.

The researchers had finally unraveled the mystery, and like all scientific mysteries, the final answer was simple because it was physical. The A, B or AB Rh-positive cells that had entered the Rh-negative mother's bloodstream through her torn and bleeding uterus were equivalent to her being given a mismatched blood transfusion, and as in any transfusion in which the blood transfused was of a different major blood group than the recipient's, the transfused cells were destroyed by antibodies already circulating in her bloodstream. The number of mismatched A, B, or AB Rh-positive cells entering the mother's body during delivery was small enough to be destroyed without causing a reaction, their destruction going on unnoticed until finally they were all gone, as if they had never been there at all.

Landsteiner had proved earlier that every person has in his

bloodstream preformed antibodies against the major blood groups other than his own. That was the reason, he had shown, for transfusion reactions in the first place. Give a person a mismatched blood type and he will have a reaction, the antibodies already in his circulation attacking the foreign red cells that are being transfused. In the cases where the Rh-negative mothers were spared, there were two incompatiabilities present: the mother was Rh-negative and her child Rh-positive, but his red cells were also of a different major blood type than her own. The anti-A or anti-B antibodies, already in her circulation, coupled to the A and B antigens on her baby's Rh-positive cells as they entered her body, and destroyed them before her immune system had the time even to recognize the Rh antigens as being there, before Rh-positive antibodies could be produced.

The researchers realized that here was the body literally using its own immune system to offset another kind of incompatibility. Defending itself with itself. It gave the researchers an idea that has become the main thrust in all of preventive modern medical research, basic or clinical. To cure a disease, not just treat it, you must help the body to do it itself. It is the body that is the hero, not science, not antibiotics, not antimetabolites, not machines or new devices. It is the body making antibodies against the swallowed polio vaccine, not the iron lungs, that cured polio. Penicillin and streptomycin may kill the majority of bacteria in an infected wound, but it is the body itself that must go after and destroy the last resistant microbe. It is the body, too, that must seek out that last single hidden cancer cell, missed by radiation therapy or methotrexate, and destroy it if the patient is to survive.

From what they had learned, the doctors reasoned that if some Rh-negative women could destroy the Rh-positive cells themselves, perhaps all women could. They also reasoned from what they had learned that perhaps there was time—not much, but enough—after delivery to get rid of any Rh-positive cells that might have entered any Rh-negative mother before she became sensitized to these cells, before she began to make the Rh-positive antibodies that would put at risk her second pregnancy.

The question had become how to do it for those Rh-negative mothers who had the same major blood group on their red cells as their Rh-positive children—in short, how to do it for all those women whose major blood group was compatible with their Rh-positive children.

It was here that the basic researchers helped by giving definitive molecular and chemical answers to what the clinicians had found. All through the forties, fifties and sixties, the basic scientists had continued their own work on antibodies. They had learned how to isolate and purify them from all the other proteins circulating in the blood. They learned how down at the molecular level these molecules worked to protect us. They were the ones who discovered how antibodies bind to antigens and how they activate complement. They also discovered, to their surprise, using pure samples of antibodies, that there were really different kinds of antibodies within the larger IgG, IgM and IgA classes, and that some of these subclasses bound complement, while others did not.

These basic scientists went on to learn how to preserve purified antibodies, the best solutions to store them in so that they could be used at a later date, how to inject them and where. All of this knowledge and technique was gradually made available to the clinical researchers. As had happened so many times before, what had once been done only in the basic researchers' labs moved to the wards. The research procedures became accepted and useful methods of clinical treatment.

The clinicians taking care of children with Rh disease began using the recently available purified IgG, which they had been told by the basic scientists contained the major anti-A, anti-B and anti-AB antibodies, as treatment. If some mothers could destroy Rh-positive cells with their own circulating anti-A and anti-B antibodies and save their future Rh-positive infants from erythroblastosis fetalis, then maybe the doctors could themselves inject anti-A or anti-B antibodies into those mothers who had none, mothers who could not destroy the Rh cells that entered their body because they were of the same major blood type as their babies.

But antibodies are blind. The doctors realized that if the mother was of the same major blood group as her Rh-positive baby, then the antibodies they injected against the baby's red cells would also go after her own.

They had the answer: destroy the Rh cells that entered the

mother at the time of delivery before she could make Rh anti-bodies. But how to do this without putting the mother herself at risk? The clinicians went back to the basic scientists. Why not forget about injecting antibodies to major blood groups, they said, and just go to the heart of the matter and inject the mother with just preformed Rh-positive antibodies? She would be pro-tected herself because her own red blood cells were Rh nega-tive; none of her red blood cells would be touched by the in-jected anti-Rh antibodies, while the Rh-positive cells of her infant that had entered her circulation would be hunted down and destroyed. And since, they reasoned, the injected Rh-posi-tive antibodies were proteins, they would, like all antibodies, gradually be destroyed by the mother's circulation, gone from her bloodstream long before her second Rh-positive child was conceived, and not be at risk himself from the injection.

The basic scientists listened. It could be done, they said. They had the technology to make the pure anti-Rh antibodies, and they did.

All the techniques of modern protein science were used. Rh-positive cells were injected into the veins of male volun-teers. Their immune system began to manufacture anti-Rh an-tibodies. Three weeks after the injection, small amounts of these volunteers' blood were removed. In an amazing combination of science, medicine and industry, the antibody fraction was sepa-rated from the removed blood, purified and concentrated so that all that was left was the Rh antibody, and this antibody was used by the clinicians for their Rh injections.

Today protection against Rh disease is routine for all Rh-negative women giving birth to Rh-positive children when the mother's major blood type is the same as that of her child. Each pregnant woman is typed during the first month of her preg-nancy. If she is found to be Rh-negative, her husband is then typed. If, as is likely, he is Rh-positive, then the infant, after he is born, is also typed. If the infant is found to be Rh-positive and of the same major blood group as the mother, a sample of her blood is assayed within a day of delivery to see if there are any Rh-positive cells in her circulation. If her baby's Rh-positive cells are found in her bloodstream, the mother is given an injec-tion of 100 micrograms of Rh antibody. These antibodies once injected search out, as if they were her own, every foreign red blood cell in her circulation of the Rh-positive type. Every Rh-positive cell that has entered her body is hunted down as if it were a microbe, a bit of poison, and destroyed. Her next child will be born healthy, and the one after that. The plague is ended.

II

Immunization: Why It Works

FOR ALL THE SEEMING MYSTERY of immunization, the DPT (diphtheria, pertussis, tetanus) series in infancy, the polio sugar cube, the measles shot, smallpox and German-measles vaccines, tetanus boosters, cholera, yellow fever, typhoid, typhus and flu shots in the end all rely on the same thing—they all rely on the ability of the body to recognize the swallowed or injected materials as foreign, and to produce antibodies against them which will from that time on always be available to protect the body if it is ever attacked again.

To use the body in this way, in a sense to artificially force it to protect itself, has been the greatest achievement of medicine. Yet it is an achievement of negatives; its success is related to things that don't happen. In this dramatic age of lifesaving implantations of cardiac pacemakers, of dying people being wheeled down hospital corridors to dialysis, of total hip replacements, open-heart surgery and corneal repairs, arterial grafts and kidney transplants, the quiet success of immunizations tends to be taken for granted.

There is none of the excitement of the emergency room or the glamour of the operating room, in not being ill; it is the medical flashes that claim our attention. Heart transplants catch the world's interest; life in a test tube becomes a cover story for *Time*. Little note is made of the fact that during the whole of World War II there was not a single case of tetanus in the entire United States Army. For the first time in history, typhus did not ravage divisions nor swamp fever leave whole regiments sick and dying, miles from the enemy. We give little thought to the fact that today civilian communities no longer suddenly flicker and go out, as so often happened in the past.

In 1664, on the island of St. Lucia in the West Indies, yellow fever killed 1,411 out of the garrison of 1,500 soldiers. The next year 200 more died of the fever; and the year after that, every man, woman and child on the island died. On Guadeloupe in 1796, out of an initial population of 20,000 the mortality rate from yellow fever was 13,807. Six years later in Santo Domingo, 27,000 Spanish troops out of its garrison of 40,000 died. In 1804 yellow fever raged through Gibraltar; of 14,000 people living there, only 28 escaped. In the Northern Hemisphere, Canada was invaded; all but six troopers of an entire English regiment stationed in Quebec died in the epidemic of 1805 and were buried there. In New Orleans from 1838 to 1883, 31,000 people died from the fever; the next largest number of deaths, fully a third less, was caused by cholera, while during that time fewer than 7,000 died from smallpox.

In 1929 a dedicated South American physician summed up in one sentence what he had learned in a lifetime of trying to treat yellow fever. "In this disease," he wrote, "toxication is everything, infection nothing or almost nothing." He was absolutely correct. Those severely affected by the fever, the hundreds of thousands who perished, indeed appeared to be poisoned. It was as if they had been stricken rather than infected. Many totally healthy were dead within three days. It had been obvious to the earliest physicians that yellow fever was not like other diseases. There was no warning, no few days of stuffy nose, no vague aches and pains, no cramps or stiffness. All the patient might experience was a very mild sense of excitement, a vague sense of anxiety, and then the disease hit.

The characteristic thing about yellow fever was always the

suddenness of its attack. In the midst of a conversation, of walking back from a barn or cutting wood, or even just talking or reading, it struck, prostratingly, blindingly, producing headaches and dizziness within seconds, fevers to 104 and 105 degrees even as the stricken person sought a place to sit down. Within hours the patient was in the grip of terrifying nausea and severe vomiting. Small children, suddenly struck, convulsed without warning.

Yet regardless of the fever the stricken patient could not sleep. Overactive and irritable, he moved about as best he could. The blinding headaches, the relentless vomiting continued. On the second day the gums would begin to ooze. On the third day the jaundice appeared. The deadly yellow color that gave the disease its name crept gradually into the stricken person's skin until even the white sclera of the eyes became a sickly, grayish yellow. With the jaundice, the vomiting of blood began. Blood turned black by the gastric juices was retched up again and again and again. So gruesome was this vomiting, so terrifying to watch that the Spaniards and Portuguese called the disease "vomito negro," the black vomit. For hundreds of years all around the world, companions, friends and family watched horrified as the stricken, burning with fever, suddenly sat bolt upright in their beds, vomited out a huge amount of black blood, collapsed and died. So brutal was yellow fever that it was as if its victims, from the time they fell ill until their final breath, had been hammered to their death, remorselessly, relentlessly battered by a combination of fever, diarrhea, headaches and vomiting until, broken, they finally died. There was no respite to any of this, no relief, no moment of comfort, just pounding, relentless, ruthless disease.

Yellow fever no longer hammers us to death and because it doesn't, it is no longer in our thoughts. We ignore it, not because the virus that causes the fever is no longer around or because the mosquitoes that transmit it are gone; they aren't. They are still both there ready to batter us again. That they don't is only because of medicine's continuing success in prevention, a success that has saved more of us than all the heart transplants, kidney machines, pacemakers and surgical procedures ever developed.

But the concern of today's medical establishment is disease.

Preventive medicine with the eloquent quietness of its achievements is taken for granted when not actually played down. It is hard, many physicians say, to get the public concerned about something that doesn't happen, or epidemics that occurred two hundred years ago, or even fifteen. Perhaps so, but if those men are right and if the ravages of yellow fever do seem too far away for us to be bothered about it, there is another disease that isn't. We can still appreciate how important preventive medicine is, how fortunate we are to have it, by taking a close look at a disease we cannot afford to ignore, one that is now preventable but is still here, awaiting its chance.

Most of us are not accustomed to think of measles as a terrifying disease; however, if it lacks the grotesqueness of yellow fever, it can be just as deadly. Perhaps it is because there is something cute about toddlers with a rash, or because so many rashes cause no problems and simply go away, that measles has come to be considered an almost off-hand disease. Mention "hepatitis" and friends are concerned; "infectious mononucleosis" and they offer support. But say "measles" and the attitude is almost a cheerful "So what?" Yet in truth, before immunization against the disease was discovered, measles was potentially as disastrous as typhus, as brutal as yellow fever.

Epidemics of measles commonly occurred in late winter or early spring at two- to four-year intervals. In the incubation stage the affected child had a slight rise in temperature. There was a day or two of being vaguely uncomfortable, then four or five of a hacking cough, runny nose and conjunctivitis. The third stage, usually severe, was ushered in on the sixth or seventh day by a sudden high fever, at times by convulsions and even bronchial pneumonia. The final stage was the rash. Even if the temperature had been high, once the rash appeared, it rose still higher. The fine red marks began first on the front of the body, the neck, along the hairline and on the posterior part of the cheeks, then rapidly within twenty-four hours, spread to cover the upper body—chest, arms, stomach—until by the third day it finally reached the feet, leaving the whole body covered. In terms of numbers, the epidemics were as grim as the epidemics of yellow fever. Virtually every susceptible person was eventually affected. It is estimated that before measles vaccinations, only 2 percent of the entire population of the United States had been spared an attack. And in terms of suffering, measles was as disastrous as the plague or smallpox.

If your child has not been immunized and has not already survived an attack of measles, he right now runs a 50 percent chance of having his brain involved during an attack. Almost one percent of those infected will not only have the rash, the cough and the high fever, but will go on to have the measles virus cause a severe and crippling encephalitis. Of these, 40 percent will survive intact, but 25 percent will have their brain destroyed, leaving them so severely retarded that if death does not intervene, the rest of their life will be spent in mental institutions among the mongoloids and hydrocephalics. The remaining 35 percent will die. Since virtually every child in America will suffer from measles, the attack rate among children being close to 100 hundred percent, the one percent number becomes meaningless. The truth is that more children have been ravaged by measles than were ever crippled by polio.

As if that weren't enough for a childhood disease most think of as innocuous, we now know that in adulthood, years after the initial attack, there can still be a desperate, late onset complication. This complication, resulting from a seemingly recovered, almost forgotten case of measles, is the subject at least once yearly of a case presentation in an infectious-disease grand rounds at every large-university medical center in the country.

"The patient you are about to see has a disease," Dr. Pierce begins before those in the auditorium have even started to settle down, "subacute sclerosing panencephalitis."

Ordinarily grand rounds provide an opportunity for the lecturer to show off a bit, to have the spotlight on his own intelligence. The lecturer knows in advance the diagnosis of the case he will be discussing and may take as long as a week or two for preparation, covering every detail of the disease, not so much to get set for the questions that will inevitably follow his presentation as to make sure there will be no questions at all. "Grand rounds" means just what it says. Unlike regular neurology rounds or hematology rounds where only a few specialists are present, the whole department of medicine comes to grand rounds to listen to what they know will be a definitive discussion of the disease under consideration. There is a muted carnival tone to it all, of knowing that you will be watching a virtuoso solo performance of case presentation. Vanity and tradition allow the lecturer to present the interesting and pertinent facts of the disease as if they had been personally discovered by him, facts usually presented in the crisp, disinterested monotone of the knowledgeable, self-assured expert totally in control of his facts.

Not this time, though. There is a gravity in Pierce's stance that cancels out the last moments of conversation and shuffling around which usually precedes the beginning of a grand rounds lecture. He is obviously not enjoying his task. His face is set, and the tone of his voice anything but disinterested.

"Lights, please," he says.

The overhead lights go out as the slide projector in the projecting booth shoots a path of hazy light down from the back of the hall.

"This first slide shows an earlier picture of the patient who will be presented here today." The photograph on the screen moves in and out until it comes into focus. "It was taken three months ago." Those in the audience see a young man standing in the midst of a group of clowning friends.

"Next."

The same young man is in a football jersey and shorts. His legs are powerful, even though in the first picture he looked slim.

"The patient is a twenty-two-year-old white male, an all-American football player, a Merit scholar; except for minor athletic injuries and an appendectomy, he had been healthy prior to the present admission. His only childhood illnesses were chicken pox, mumps and measles. The next picture was taken only two months ago."

It is the same young man, this time with his arm around a lovely dark-haired girl. They are standing by a motorcycle, smiling at whoever is taking the snapshot.

"According to the boy's parents," Pierce continues, "the attack of childhood measles lasted approximately nine days. They are good historians and remembered the three or four days of coughing and conjunctivitis followed by a high fever and the typical measles rash." The photograph stays on; the young man's personable smile beaming down off the large screen seems out of place in the heavy austerity of the semidark auditorium. "There was no evidence of encephalopathy. The parents state that their son gradually recovered from his attack of measles; no seizures; there was no listlessness other than that associated with the high fever. The rash gradually faded. He recovered within a week and was back at school in two. He had been healthy until this admission.

"Next."

A photograph of a hospital bed flashes on the screen. In the bed is an emaciated young man, the same young man as in the previous photographs, though hardly recognizable.

"Next."

The bedcover has been removed and the photograph shows the patient, head thrown back, thin arms rigidly twisted out in front of his body, ending in the clawlike hands of decerebrate rigidity. There is a restless stirring in the audience—a few lean forward to get a better look. "What did he say the dates were?" someone asks in the dark.

"Lights," the doctor requests.

The overhead lights spring on. Pierce nods to the intern and the resident sitting in the front row near the side exit. The two men rise and walk quietly up the three steps to the podium stage and then out the side door.

"Subacute sclerosing panencephalitis is now known to be one of the late complications of measles," Pierce says. "It has been reported as early as three years after the initial measles attack and as late as twenty. And its course, once begun—" The side door opens and everybody turns to look. The intern, backing in, holds open the door to let the resident roll in the wheelchair. "—is rapid and progressive."

The young man of the last two photographs is wheeled in, a rope tied around his chest. Unconscious, he hangs forward in the chair. As he is being rolled across the stage his head, drooped against his chest, begins to slowly twitch and then to convulse from side to side. His bony hands clench and unclench while his arms, limp at his side, jerk about as if pulled by a malicious puppeteer.

Pierce keeps silent as the resident pauses in the center of the stage to turn the wheelchair so that the helpless patient faces the audience. Even as those in the auditorium watch in shocked silence, the patient throws back his head and with his eyes staring blindly up at the lighted ceiling, lets out a shriek so unexpected and so terrifying that many, despite all their professionalism, shrink back. It takes a while for the room to settle down.

They are not used to seeing the severely retarded. They have come expecting the sharp briskness of a medical discussion on an infectious disease, the preciseness of antibiotic levels and dosages, drug absorptions and clearance rates. They have expected to witness medicine at its cleanest and at its best—the comforting definiteness of bacterial cultures being read out as 100,000 colonies per cc. or 50,000, of smears being positive or negative. Now they are forced into a nervous and uneasy silence by the very thing they are supposedly trained to deal with—illness. All of us have to learn, doctor or truck driver, to recognize the hazards of being human; indeed, it is familiarity with those hazards that makes control possible, and nowhere is that effort at control more stringently pursued and more actively practiced than in medicine. It is a control geared to containment, to maintaining order. But every now and then even to physicians the truth breaks through—what illness really means, and the price that is paid for it in human suffering.

The resident and intern who had wheeled the poor young man onto the stage stand grimly by the wheelchair. In the uneasy silence pervading the room, you can feel the relief when Pierce at last nods to the two men to remove the patient.

"The patient you have just seen," he says, turning back to those in the auditorium, "was perfectly healthy until two months ago. At that time he began experiencing emotional lability; almost overnight he began crying at nothing, or rather, everything. His friends thought it was the pressure of school. Within days he stopped going to classes, he let his work fall off, he began picking fights. In one of these fights he was severely beaten. His fiancée, who was with him at the time, explained that he didn't strike back even though he had begun the fight. She stated that he did not seem to be able to protect himself, that apparently he didn't see or simply couldn't get out of the way of his attackers once he had provoked them. The beating necessitated an emergency-room visit at the county hospital. During the examination an alert physician noticed severe incoordination out of proportion to his injuries. The patient was told of this finding, its implications, but refused to be admitted. Two days later he was again brought into that emergency room, this time convulsing and in *status epilepticus.*

"That was five weeks ago," Pierce continues. "I will not go through the differential diagnosis of seizure disorders. That would not be appropriate for this type of grand rounds, but I will say that *status epilepticus,* continuous seizures, can deplete the brain cells of necessary nutrients and cause brain damage in itself. We have not, as you have seen, even after four weeks of treatment been able to stop the patient's seizures. This type of picture—impaired intellect, personality problems, emotional lability, incoordination, seizures with rapid mental deterioration, plus characteristic bursts of slow waves on EEG combined with retinal degeneration and blindness—is not unfamiliar.

"At autopsy, patients with this constellation of symptoms show either a rapidly expanding brain tumor or a bizarre pathological process that has been termed subacute sclerosing panencephalitis. In the latter condition the post-mortem examination of the brain shows only dead and dying brain cells replaced by scar tissue. In these patients there is no evidence on brain sections of any tumor whatsoever—nor is there any clinical evidence of a brain tumor with the patient you have just seen. The cause of this degenerative process was formerly unknown, but recently, with the use of new immunological techniques and viral cultures, the cause has been found.

"Dawson in the early forties, doing autopsies on patients such as these, noticed that in their degenerating brain cells were what he called inclusion bodies—tiny structures found in some, but not in all sections of the examined brain-cell nuclei. It was thought at first that these particles were nothing more than degenerating subnuclear particles and later that they might in fact be viruses, but the virus theory was never proved because no viruses could ever be grown from these biopsy samples or from fresh brain autopsy specimens. The disease has since that time been called interchangeably Dawson's inclusion body encephalitis and subacute sclerosing panencephalitis.

"With our new immunological techniques, we now know that these patients, like the patient just presented, have very high concentrations of measles antibodies in their spinal fluid. Recently, with our new viral tissue-culture technique, we have been able to grow a virus from these patients' brains—a virus proved to be identical to the wild measles virus itself.

"We assume today that the inclusion particles that Dawson saw in the sections of brain in the patients he biopsied over twenty years ago were indeed aggregated portions of the measles virus itself."

Pierce hestiates, and then, looking around the room, pronounces the sentence. "There have been no reported cases of recurring measles; one attack supposedly gives lifelong immunity. With this knowledge we can only postulate that the measles viruses found in the brain of a patient with subacute sclerosing panencephalitis have been there, lying dormant, ever since the original attack of measles. For some unknown reason these viruses, inactive in the patient's brain cells, absolutely quiescent, begin to grow again as late as twenty years after the original infection, destroying the cells in which they had obviously lain dormant for so long. It is equally obvious that during this period the patient's body ignored these viruses, or else after the initial childhood attack the viruses inside the brain cells were so adequately shielded from the body's defenses that the patient's immune system could never reach them.

"The body's immune system obviously destroyed most of the originally invading measles viruses, but some, getting into a few of the brain cells, were able—why we don't know—to hide there and survive. When they begin—again for what reason we don't know—to grow in the cells where they have been harbored for so long, the body's immune system responds. In an effort to destroy the growing viruses—or at least to wall them off and keep them from infecting other brain cells—the infected brain is flooded with antibodies, lymphocytes, white cells, complement and properdin. In the melee that follows, infected cells and normal cells are destroyed together. The immune reaction is so severe, the reaction mounted against these destructive viruses so powerful that vessels, connective tissues and healthy brain cells in the immediate area of the battle are themselves injured.

"In most cases an immune response is lifesaving—because the infecting organism is usually controlled, with only small amounts of normal tissues themselves being destroyed in the process. But unlike liver or kidney tissue, which can regenerate, or muscle cells that can be lost without concern, a brain cell once destroyed is destroyed forever. It doesn't matter; virus or immune reaction, once a brain cell begins to degenerate it is gone and can never be replaced; once it dies, that part of the circuit is out—and out forever. In the case of a viral brain disease, the body's own defenses once brought into play only add to the neuronal destruction being caused by the virus, and account in large part itself for the patient's rapid deterioration from seeming normality to sudden emotional lability, physical disability and death, often without coma or unconsciousness, sometimes within weeks. Once the infectious viral process begins and the immune response is mounted, there is no cure, no medication, no hope.

"We have all had measles," Pierce concludes. "We have each, supposedly, recovered. And yet . . ."

After the rounds are over, there are comments about the inappropriateness of his warning as well as his bringing in the patient. Some say that he got too involved; others complain that personal statements, much less warnings, have no place at grand rounds, that in fact there is no medical reason to have actually brought in that kind of patient in the first place or for that matter any kind of patient into an infectious-disease grand rounds. Yet there is not one person leaving the lecture hall who does not at some time during that day at least for a moment wonder, since they have all had measles, if he or she, too, might not, by some trick of fate—some defect in his own immunity, a chance unexplainable occurrence some years before—still have the original measles virus lodged somewhere in his own brain, ready in a week or two or a month to suddenly, for reasons beyond his control, begin to grow again.

If that happens—and it will happen somewhere to someone, as it always has—it will be for no other reason than that the victim was born too late to be immunized.

TODAY MEASLES, like yellow fever, should hold no terror for anyone; no one born into this age need ever again be pushed unconscious and twitching out onto a medical podium. No one ever again should have to leave a conference or walk down a hallway wondering if perhaps his own brain will soon be destroyed.

Yellow fever was not cured by Walter Reed; his companions and his friends did not die in a battle to wipe out the disease, but to control its spread. The cure had to await the yellow-fever vaccine. It was the development of the attenuated 17-D strain of the yellow-fever arbovirus that eliminated the disease once and for all from the world.

Similarly with measles, those children inoculated with the Edmonston strain of the attenuated live measles virus vaccine are protected not only from the encephalitis that can result from the original measles attack but it appears, also from the late, though equally terrifying complication of sclerosing panencephalitis.

And so it goes with polio and German measles, too, with typhoid and typhus, cholera, plague, smallpox, rubella, rabies and Rocky Mountain spotted fever. Vaccines work because when we get our shots, when we are vaccinated, when we swallow the live attenuated strain of the wild polio virus, things happen within us that are as basic as the universe, as real and substantial as the oceans we swim in and the earth we walk on. There is wisdom in that happening, and great wizardry, but it is an earthy wizardry and at best a brutal wisdom gained not through thought or science, but through a billion years of our body's relentless struggle for its own survival.

That knowledge, all of it, is our heritage bequeathed to us by an ancestry that would not give up; it is a wisdom paid for by countless trials and errors, by terrible mistakes and blunders. Now that final finished process is ours, full blown and monumental, a present to each and every one of us. It is the recognition of this inheritance that has made it possible for a few men working alone, without doctrine or support, often scoffed at and ridiculed, to save us from the ravages of so many diseases, and may yet someday save us from cancer as well.

•   •   •

THE BASIC IDEA at the center of all immunological research, of immunization itself, is to let the body do it, to help the body do it, to use the body's own massive resources to cure and heal itself. Like all great ideas, this one is incredibly simple. But in practice, it has taken well over a hundred years of effort and work, frustration and courage, to prove its worth and make it generally applicable.

The whole idea of immune defense has nothing to do with the romantic notion of the body killing things, of being able to sense the malevolence of attacking microbes and then going after them. Rather, it rests on the blindness of chemical evolution, in the beginning when molecules began competing and then later when one cell type started distinguishing and destroying another. The theory of immunization—what Pasteur and Jenner did by injecting materials into people's bodies—depends first and foremost on a property that developed early in the struggles of those primeval seas: the ability of one cell to recognize a cell which was unlike itself.

Individual recognition had to precede individual destruction, and that recognition, from the beginnings of cellular evolution on, depended on surfaces. After the processes that gave rise to life began to be assembled behind the protection of membranes, the killing began. One cell attacked the other, using the chemical differences in their cellular surface to distinguish like from unlike. Once a cell had identified another as "foreign," as being different, the attack began; the sugars, fats and amino acids locked up inside the loser becoming available as food to the conqueror.

As life became more and more complicated and self-sufficient and as its internal machinery increased in size and complexity, the number of its chemical parts—the compounds, carrier proteins, enzymes, coenzymes, genes, operons, minerals and salts necessary to maintain the ever more efficient life processes—multiplied, as did the defenses necessary to protect them. Chemical poisons evolved, cellular capsules and coats developed, cell walls thickened, but then as now, the membrane, the outer surface of an organism, continued to be used as the identifier. The different arrangement of the molecules and compounds in these surfaces—the antigens—are still used, as they were in those first seas and as they are now within our own bodies, to start the whole reaction of cellular attack and immune defense.

Outer cellular membranes have always been structurally sound, rigid walls that provide not only protection for cells but support as well. In many ways these membranes that surround every cell, even the cells of our own bodies, are much like the plastic casing covering your telephone—a hard outer shell protecting the delicate internal circuits—or like the walls of your house protecting the people and things within. The plastic telephone casings or the brick walls, like the membranes around all cells, are made up of inert materials that once put together are not easily destroyed. A house may be gutted on the inside, but the walls or parts of them will still stand. The inside of the phone may short-circuit and burn, but the outer casing, even if warped from the heat, remains.

It is the same in nature. A cell may be killed or a bacterium destroyed, but its cell walls made of the inert solid polymers of protein continue to exist. When cells die, their outer membranes can still be seen under the microscope, ghostly hollow shapes floating around with nothing inside. Partially intact, like the warped, burned outer casing of a useless phone or the standing walls of a gutted house, they can still be recognized for what they were. In the same way, the outer bacterial coats of dead organisms, when injected into the body, are recognized by the body's immune system for what they were and the whole immune response is activated, as if these foreign bits and pieces of bacterial cell walls were still surrounding a living dangerous organism. The body responds only to surfaces; it doesn't have time to check or wait to see if the surface is part of something that is alive or dead; it cannot take the chance. The battle for life has always been fought surface against surface, but with the injection of dead organisms the battle cannot be lost. The body always wins.

This is why immunizations work. Pasteur eliminated anthrax as a plague of animals by culturing the anthrax organisms, killing them in a test tube with formalin, grinding up the whole mess and injecting it into susceptible cows and sheep that would have contracted the disease. The anthrax bacteria he injected were dead, and being dead, could not multiply in the animals' bodies, could not cause the disease. But the bacteria walls were still intact, and once the animals' immune system was exposed to these walls, and the antigens on their surface were read as foreign, antibodies were produced against them.

During later epidemics, when the live anthrax bacillus did indeed attack these previously injected animals, antibodies developed against the previously injected dead organisms were already circulating in their bodies, and these went right after the invading organisms. The membranes this time surrounded live bacteria, they were "holed" by circulating anti-anthrax antibodies and the animals' complement system, and the live bacteria were destroyed before they could multiply and cause disease. It is this fact and this fact alone, that it is the outside of organisms, their membranes—whether bacteria, viruses or fungi—our immune system responds to, and not the living organisms within, which makes all vaccinations possible, indeed has made them work.

It is this fact that is the center pillar of all immunologic thought and research, and now lies at the very heart of the newest theory of cancer growth—immune surveillance. All the supposedly complex ideas of immunology, of immune disorders, of resistance and immune tolerance, even of immune surveillance, can be understood by just remembering this one fact: the body will respond to the antigens in foreign cell walls, whether they surround a live cell or a dead one. It is how Pasteur, Jenner, Enders, Sabin, Robbins and Salk were able to succeed.

THERE ARE TODAY two major types of vaccines, those that contain dead microbes and those that contain live ones. Pasteur's anthrax vaccine was the first use of a bacterial vaccine containing dead microbes; Jenner's vaccine against smallpox the first use of a viral vaccine containing live organisms. But it was Pasteur's technical achievement in the development of the rabies vaccine which led the way to the development of all modern-day viral vaccines.

For the rabies vaccine Pasteur again used a dead microbe —but with a difference. At the time he developed the vaccine he had no idea what caused rabies. Like others, he looked at the saliva of rabid dogs, expecting to find the rabies bacillus there, but found nothing. Yet when he took that same saliva and injected it into normal animals, they developed rabies just as surely and just as quickly as if they had actually been bitten by a rabid dog.

Pasteur took the investigation of the saliva one step further. Using a very fine porcelain filter, he poured the saliva over the top of it. Any particle, any bit of matter the size of a bacterium or larger would not be able to pass through the fine pores of the porcelain. But when the filtered saliva was injected, it still caused rabies in the injected animals. It was clear to Pasteur that the infective agent was there in the filtered saliva and remained 100 percent lethal. Whatever caused rabies, it was not bacteria; they would have been too big not to have been seen under the microscope or to have passed through the filter.

He made another observation. Today it seems obvious and perhaps even trite, but then, working alone, with no guidance, with only his previous discovery or preceding observation to go on, having no theory to fit any of it together and trusting only in the scientific method, Pasteur made a discovery that was crucial not only to those bitten by rabid animals but to the rest of humanity as well, indeed to every living thing.

By letting the saliva dry on the microscope slide and then injecting the dried material, Pasteur found it was no longer infectious. He could let the saliva dry and scrape it off the slide and inject it into healthy animals and the animal would not become ill, would not acquire rabies. Whatever it was that was in the saliva, whatever it was that couldn't be seen or filtered, it was no longer there when the saliva was dried—or else it had died. Using the filter, he tested the blood and other tissue fluids of rabid animals as he had their saliva and found the infective agent in their brain as well, which was not surprising, since the symptoms of the rabid animals were all related to a maddened, disease-ridden nervous system. Pasteur wondered if by drying these infected brains he could do to them what he had done with the saliva—kill the infective agent, then take the dried brain, hopefully no longer infectious, and by reinjecting it into healthy animals protect them as he had protected the cows and sheep from anthrax. It worked, and not only with dogs and cats but with humans as well.

What Pasteur did in protecting against rabies by injecting the dried brains of rabid animals is what is done when you or your child is given a shot for smallpox, measles, mumps, German

[141]

measles, influenza, typhus, typhoid, whooping cough or yellow fever. The dead or modified microbe is injected directly into the body. The cell walls of the microbe, even if the microbe is dead or slightly different from the disease-causing organism—as in the case of the virus in the smallpox and measles vaccine—can no longer cause disease but are still structurally intact, still antigenic. With the microbial walls intact, our body responds to the injection as if the organism was still dangerous. Antibodies are made, complement is utilized, T and B lymphocytes are stimulated, white cells are marshaled and thrown forward toward the nonexistent threat. Eventually the small number of the injected noninfectious, though antigenic organisms are broken down, eliminated from the body, and the immune system relaxes. But having once been stimulated, it is now totally alerted.

Small amounts of antibody, specific for the injected organisms, continue forever to move about in the circulation, while stimulated lymphocytes, triggered for any return of the microbe used in the immunization, patrol the vessels—ready for the next time the body is attacked, the next time the same foreign membrane shows itself. And that next time it will be the live microbes attacking in force, trying to cause disease.

But the body now has the advantage; because of its previous immunization, it is able to destroy the attackers before they can even get a foothold. Preformed antibodies and lymphocytes instantaneously available now destroy the attacking microbes in the area where they have entered the body, before they can multiply, before they can spread out or go deeper into the vital organs. A previously immunized person can stop the invasion on the beaches, wipe out the enemy before it can even begin to gather itself for any real assault.

WE KNOW NOW what Pasteur did not: that rabies is caused by a virus, a microbe many times smaller than a bacterium, impossible to be seen under the light microscope, and able to pass through the finest filters. As a scourge, it was eliminated by Pasteur's rabies vaccine, by antibodies also too small to be seen, also able to pass through the finest filters, actually themselves one-hundredth the size of the rabies virus. The antibodies protect those bitten by rabid animals by coating the walls of the invading viruses, keeping them from adhering to the cells of the body, from getting into the nerves and from there into the brain, where the viruses would have slowly multiplied, causing disease and horrible death.

Smallpox too is caused by a virus, and what Jenner accomplished with his smallpox immunization was exactly what Pasteur achieved with his anthrax and rabies shots, but he used a live virus, one similar to the smallpox virus but slightly different.

Unlike Pasteur, Jenner did not attack the problem of disease with the tools and methods of science. He was a simple country doctor, a clinician, an observer of people, of suffering and disease. What he did was no more than to observe that people who worked closely with cows could and did occasionally contract cowpox, and after a day or two of low-grade fever and a few smallpox-like postules, they would recover and from then on be resistant to smallpox. The observation gave him an idea and he began a clinical experiment, without benefit of test tubes, laboratory or rigorous scientific method. He simply took the pus from the cowpox lesion on a cow, scratched it onto people's arms and watched to see if they would contract smallpox. They didn't. His immunized patients were as protected from smallpox as Pasteur's were to be from rabies.

Today we know the why of both. The principles involved in both types of immunization—the use of live viruses as well as dead ones—are exactly the same, even though the methods employed are different. Pasteur injected a dead virus whose outer coat was still intact. Jenner scratched onto the skin a live virus whose outer covering happened to be so similar antigenically to the disease-causing smallpox virus that once the cowpox was injected into humans, an antibody response was mounted that would cross-react with the smallpox virus, and so protect the immunized person from the ravages of that disease.

There is some indication that the cowpox virus is related to the smallpox virus, that millions of years ago the pox viruses split —the cowpox adapting itself to hoofed animals, the smallpox to the primates. But parts of their membranes, a few antigens, remained similar, showing their common heritage, and it is this similarity, this common antigenicity, that leads to cowpox protecting us. When the rather mild virus is scratched onto our skin, our immune system responds, making antibodies, stimulating lymphocytes, organizing its white cells, and because the cowpox virus is not adapted to humans, it is easily destroyed, quickly eliminated from the body. But the immune response is then geared not only for a reattack of the cowpox virus but for an attack of the antigenically similar but far more deadly small-pox virus. The cowpox antibodies will go after the smallpox viruses, destroying them as soon as they attack, before they can cause even one pox, before the person attacked even begins to feel the beginning of the disease. It is the same with all immuni-zations.

For over a hundred and fifty years the use of a live preven-tive vaccine had been limited to the utilization of the cowpox virus to protect us against smallpox. Jenner's finding was incred-ible good luck for mankind; all one has to do is read about the suffering and high death rate of the seventeenth- and eight-eenth-century smallpox plagues of Paris and London to under-stand this. Men continually looked and hoped for that kind of luck again but couldn't find it. There were, of course, other seemingly similar diseases in both men and animals, but either the animal virus was so markedly different from the human virus that it would not grow in man or the diseases were so similar, perhaps even the same, that the inoculations took too well, giving the injected persons the feared and deadly disease itself. One by one the bacterial plagues were conquered, but the viral plagues continued. Cowpox remained the only naturally occurring animal disease which, when injected into a human, would protect him from the human scourge. To control the other diseases, men had to look to themselves, to their own ingenuity.

The ideas of how to vaccinate were all there; Pasteur had done it for rabies, yet each year polio continued to leave thou-sands of normal children crippled and broken, measles turned thousands more into idiots, yellow fever continued to smother community after community, congenital rubella relentlessly struck down fetus after fetus, leaving each year tens of hundreds of infants blinded, microcephalic and brain-damaged. The terri-ble sufferings went on: newborn after newborn ruined, children forced to crawl when they should have been able to run, adoles-cents stumbling blindly about feeling for door handles they should have been able to see, family after family stricken.

Physicians, helpless, continued to witness it all, but there were some who refused to accept the suffering and set about to do for the other viral plagues what had already been done for smallpox and rabies. It was a continuous struggle of more than a hundred years, a century-long series of failures, and the price for each failure in terms of human life and grief too great even to begin to calculate. It was with this price in mind that the researchers toiled on.

They tried as Pasteur had done to make dead vaccines, killing with chemicals or heat what they thought were the unseen infectious organisms and injecting the supposedly dead microbes into healthy people. But that didn't work. Even later, when the researchers succeeded in isolating the infecting virus, they still couldn't seem to kill them. The acids, heat or poisons that easily killed bacteria, or indeed any other living thing, did not seem to touch these microbes. Even after being boiled or treated with phenol, they still, when injected as vaccines, continued to cause the disease.

The problem was the viruses themselves. Even today there is much argument as to exactly what a virus is, but there is no argument as to what it is made of. Experiment after experiment has shown that a virus is composed of two parts, an outer inert protein shell that surrounds and seemingly protects a soft inner core of a very special molecule, DNA, named for the chemicals that are linked together to make it up: nucleic acid, the sugar desoxyribose, and molecules of oxygen and phosphate—or sometimes a slight variation of the DNA called RNA.

DNA is the chemical substance, the polymer that all scientists agree carries the genetic code. It may very well have been the first polymer formed in the seas where life began; it is probably the actual beginnings of life, the first compound that could reproduce itself and then, as the struggle for chemical survival continued to mount, directed the production of other, smaller polymers. In the course of evolution the DNA polymer took up the central position in the nucleus of the newly forming cells. It acted, then as now, as overall master coordinator of cellular function, making sure through its molecular code that each cell's enzymes and compounds were manufactured when they were supposed to be at the right times and in the correct amounts to keep the cell healthy and through that health the entire body functioning and protected.

We know today that all living things contain the chemical compound DNA. It is the prerequisite for life. In humans it forms the nuclear chromosomes that make up our genes, deciding through the genetic control of cellular enzymes exactly how we are formed, what we are, and what we might be.

Difficult as it may be to believe, the differences in all living things have only to do with differences in the specific arrangement and sequence of the chemicals that make up their DNA. Its general helical structure, whether in plants or animals, remains the same throughout the living world, a common heritage coming from the same common beginnings.

12

Immunization: How It Works

EVERY VIRUS contains DNA, or its variant polymer RNA, yet in the laboratory it is anything but alive; indeed, observed by themselves, outside of the cells they infect, viruses appear to be dead. This was the second problem that faced the scientists trying to make viral vaccine; not only couldn't they seem to kill the viruses once they had isolated them but they couldn't, using any of the known biological nutrients, get them to grow either. They could get bacteria to divide, and fungi, parasites, single-celled organisms of all kinds could be made to multiply, but not viruses.

And so the confusion. Containing the polymer DNA, a chemical found only in living things, they seemed anything but alive; indeed, taken from the body and looked at under the microscope, they not only appeared but were absolutely inert. And yet they were obviously infective, able to multiply and cause disease when injected back into the human body. The question remained for decades whether viruses were alive or dead.

Today we realize they hold a middle ground. Outside the body, a virus is nonliving—just a tiny crystalline structure, appearing under the electron microscope as nothing more than a minute, sharply etched piece of silica or particle of quartz. It might as well be a piece of organic debris picked off the moon, to be examined here on earth. There is no vibration in it, nor any flowing. It does not consume oxygen, it does not divide, it does not grow, nor it does not move.

All of life, even the experiments that have come close to developing life in a test tube, have one thing in common— movement, if manifested only as energy being used up or transferred. To maintain life and the intricacies of its processes, energy must be utilized. The smallest, most primitive cell at rest or even dying, when placed in a scientific metabolic chamber, will continue to consume almost undetectable but still measurable amounts of oxygen. But a virus placed in the same chamber does nothing. There is no transfer of heat, no oxygen is used, no radiation given off or absorbed. For all practical purposes, outside the body it is dead, an inert polymer of DNA, lying within an inert protein sheath and so, since seemingly already dead, impossible to kill.

Outside the body the virus that causes hepatitis can survive being heated to over 140 degrees F. for an hour or freezing to −70 degrees. It can resist acids and alkalis, be placed in corrosive ammonia and phenol solutions, and still, after all this, when placed back under the electron microscope, just sit there virtually unchanged, no more affected by the battering than a piece of diamond might be. And yet, when it is injected back into the body, it can again cause hepatitis.

Something happens to that virus when it is reinjected into the body and re-enters liver cells. Oxygen suddenly begins to be consumed by the infected cell, heat is given off, energy is transferred and utilized as the virus comes gradually to life.

There are forces in nature that we not only don't understand but whose existence we are unaware of. In the late nineteenth century the physicists were convinced there was nothing left to discover. Optics, mechanics, hydrodynamics had all been worked out. A few finishing touches on some of the new ideas like electricity, and it was felt that all the mysteries of the world would be solved. But then Röntgen, by chance, left a key on a piece of newly discovered unexposed photographic film which he had placed near a large piece of uranium-containing rock. When he went to use the film he found it ruined, fogged over, while the key sitting on top of the photographic surface had left its silhouette etched onto the film. A new force, one that had always been there, was finally discovered, and the world of classical physics fell apart under the strain of trying to explain Röntgen's discovery, of dealing with a force that came out of solid rock, that acted at a distance and could with no apparent effort leave the imprint of metal objects on photographic surfaces.

Today we are a bit like those nineteenth-century physicists, if perhaps not quite so arrogant. As of now, we have no idea what turns a virus on, what force it senses that comes only from living cells. There is a feeling among virologists groping for an answer that whatever that force is, it must be chemical, that there is something about a living cell, something on its surface, a chemical substance in it, exuded by it, or something in the very nature of life itself, that suddenly triggers the inert virus and brings it to life, that starts it reproducing itself.

But if we don't know what turns viruses on, we know at least what happens once they begin to grow. Most of our present knowledge of how viruses work comes from elegant electron microscopic studies done on infected tissues. We know, because we can now see that these lifeless particles, when they come into contact with human tissue, suddenly stick to the surface of the tissue's cells. It is the first step in their reproduction, and the beginning of viral disease.

For viruses, the sticking is not a generalized occurrence, but an amazingly specific one; certain viruses will stick only to specific cells. The rabies virus, because of its own peculiarities, sticks only to nerve cells; the hepatitis virus only to liver. Those that cause encephalitis circulate throughout the body grabbing on only to brain cells; those that cause carditis, only to the heart. You can see on the electron micrographs of diseased tissues how once the virus attaches itself to a cell, its outer viral coat comes to life and pushes out a little part of itself which acts as a tiny knife cutting through the cell's wall. Once through, the viral coat that seemed so dead begins mysteriously to pulsate, to contract, pushing the DNA of its central inner core out into the interior of the cell itself.

Then occurs one of the most astonishing and deadly events in all of nature. It might be called disease, but in reality it is nothing more than chemical robbery—an example of the vicious chemical struggles that preceded life and have always been a part of it. The viral DNA injected into the human cell begins to take over the cell's inner machinery. The human DNA sitting in the nucleus, which normally directs the cell, is short-circuited, somehow suppressed, while the invading DNA begins to redirect all the cell's enzymes and polymers to begin to manufacture not the proteins and hormones that the cell usually produces and the body needs, but more viral DNA like itself and more protein coats like the one it left sticking to the outside of the cell. In the course of hours, thousands of new viruses are born, the infected cell becomes full of these new viral particles and then, dying, bursts open, releasing the newly formed particles to infect other cells where the robbery begins all over again. Within days, brains can be destroyed; hepatitis produced; the heart muscle cells so weakened that heart failure and heart attacks occur; peripheral nerve cells taken over, causing polio and death.

This process of viral thievery has been going on almost since time began—until men decided to stop it. The tenacity with which viruses took over living cells was the same tenacity with which they remained dead once outside the body. If their inertness outside of tissues is an adaptive mechanism, a way of keeping safe when not reproducing, of protecting themselves against the dangers of the world, it has proved astonishingly successful. Scientists tried continually to grow them in cultures, but it was obvious that if the virus needed some force to turn it on, it was a force connected only with living cells. You simply could not spread a virus on a nutrient broth, as you could other microbes, and have it grow. One by one the bacterial and fungal plagues were conquered, but the viral diseases went on.

During the time efforts were being made to grow viruses, medicine continued to progress. Antibodies were discovered, 30-percent-burn victims no longer died, heart valves damaged from rheumatic fever began to be replaced, coronary by-pass became routine, but polio and measles continued to ravage the young, hepatitis still felled those who contracted it, and German measles went on crossing placentas, mutilating infants even before they were born. For all the new-found sophistication of clinical medicine, despite all the isolation and culture techniques of the bacteriologists, the immunologists' own increasing understanding of allergy and infections, the final answer to the viral plagues had nothing to do with anything any of them knew. It came, rather, from another group of men, working in another area, out at the very borders of science, trying to do what had never been done before.

So seemingly erudite was their work that friends and colleagues questioned of what possible use it could be, wondering why anyone would waste his time on such a project. Yet what these basic researchers had taken upon themselves, like Pasteur and Jenner before them, was a seemingly impossible task, but one that would in time form the full answer to measles and mumps, become the cure for yellow fever and rubella. Their discovery would, within fifteen years, be the single most important tool used to conquer the viral plagues; it would be used to dismantle the iron lung, to end finally after a million years the horrible summers of recurrent paralysis and slow death.

Three pediatricians, Robbins, Enders and Weller, working at Harvard and having nothing to do with immunology or even infectious disease, tried simply to see if they could take normal animal tissues and grow them outside the body in nothing more than an artificial culture media. They started with monkey liver and kidney cells, but it was not an easy task. Carefully removing the organs from the animals, they sectioned them into thin sheets, and laying the sheets along the bottom of sterile culture dishes, immersed them in various basic nutrient broths. The tissues died. The three men tried other broths, and still the tissues died—and continued to die. One failure was followed by the next, but the researchers refused to give up; through years of laborious, tedious trial and error they learned how correctly to prepare the tissues, how to cut them down to only one-cell layers of thickness. They found that animal or human serum was essential, discovered the correct amount of vitamins to add to the broths, the precise concentration of serum proteins, the necessary antibiotics, the correct concentrations of oxygen, carbon dioxide and nitrogen, the proper amount of sugars, the right numbers of amino acids, the exact fat concentrations, the optimum temperatures to sustain the tissues' growth in the sterile dishes.

What they learned, bit by bit, was to do for the tissues all the things the body did for them while they were still in place inside the animal. It had been a grueling task taking years, but with the discovery of how to grow live cells artificially in culture media, no one need ever again live in fear of being crippled by polio or retarded by measles, parents no longer have to be worried about their child being born blind because of congenital rubella. The ability to grow cells in culture was the one single discovery immunologists needed to produce viral vaccines. They had known for years that viruses had to have living cells to grow, and now, because of the tenacity of these three pediatricians, there were billions of cells available in which to grow viruses that for so long had been ungrowable.

Yellow fever fell, then influenza, then polio, then measles, then German measles, and mumps, and soon chickenpox. Both Salk and Sabin used tissue-culture methods to grow the polio virus for their vaccines. Enders himself, applying his own techniques, developed the measles vaccine.

By the late sixties, using the viral isolation and culture methods he had been laboring over for a third of his life, Enders was finally able to grow the wild measles virus that he had cultured from the throat of a severely ill child by the name of Edmonston who was suffering from measles. Of all the viruses, the measles virus is the most fastidious in its growth demands. But Enders was able to have it grow in his tissue cultures. He watched through his microscope as the wild measles viruses, multiplying, slowly destroyed the kidney-tissue cells lying at the bottom of his culture dish. Taking the wild viruses he had grown, he injected them into monkeys, the only species other than man susceptible to measles infection. The monkeys became ill.

Enders waited days for the disease to get a good hold and then, taking blood samples from the monkeys—in a sense harvesting the wild viruses from their blood—inoculated them out into his tissue cultures and watched again as the viruses slowly destroyed the tissue cells. What he was looking for was a change in the destructiveness of the wild virus. The theory from the time of Pasteur—indeed, which Pasteur had proved with his first chicken cholera vaccine—was that microbes grown in other than their original hosts were forced to change, that their new and unfamiliar environment forced adaptive changes in the microbes themselves, just as any changing environment causes adaptive changes in any living thing. The hope was that by being able to culture and grow the wild human measles viruses and then grow them in monkeys—a different environment than the human tissues they had adapted to—these viruses, like Pasteur's cholera bacteria, would change and the change would show up first in a decreased infectivity of the tissue-culture cells.

After many passes of the original Edmonston viruses through one monkey after another, Enders began to notice less injury in the tissue cultures. The viruses no longer seemed to spread as quickly from cell to cell. Then, after a few more passes through yet more monkeys, there was no destruction at all; the tissue-culture cells continued to thrive, even though Enders could prove the viruses were still there in the broth that bathed the cells. The wild measles virus had been changed—"attenuated."

Enders, with measles, and Salk before him with the polio virus, had accomplished in their laboratories what nature had done with the cowpox virus over millions of years. They had changed the wild virus but still had it retain enough similarity to the original parent that when the attenuated strain was injected into the human body, only a mild disease would develop, yet the antibodies produced by the injection of the attenuated strain would be effective against the wild virus too. They would be there to protect those who were vaccinated when the wild virus tried to infect them.

It took Enders a few more years to be sure the attenuated Edmonston strain of the wild measles virus would not revert back to the wild type, that when injected into people, it would continue to cause the appropriate antibody production and in adequate amounts to insure against any future measles infection, without causing diseases itself.

Edmonston is the name now printed on every vial of measles vaccine. It is a name that means the end of a scourge which had covered the earth since mankind began.

· · ·

OUR BATTLES for survival have been not only against bacteria and viruses; but from the very beginning, we have had to fight poisons, too. Indeed, poisons were our earliest enemies; we fought them long before there was a single bacterium, long before the first virus was formed. Even as life was first developing, the lands too were forming. Rain drained off the new-formed continents, carrying into the warm coastal waters tons of dissolved iron, zinc, cobalt, magnesium and copper. For the cells developing in those waters, the new metals flowing into the seas around them and getting into their chemical machinery were as poisonous as the arsenic or DDT of today. In defense, cells bound those metallic atoms to their proteins and to their fats. Those cells survived that were better able to bind those metals within them, that developed compounds with greater affinity to hold them, so that once inside the cell, the poisons could be tightly bound up—were neutralized—before they could go on to disrupt the cell's chemistry. In the millions of years that followed, those metals, now inside the surviving cells but neutralized by them, became a stable part of intracellular life and later were used in a controlled way by those same cells as catalytic agents to speed up the newer, more efficient energy processes.

The atom of iron that today lies at the center of the hemoglobin molecule and binds the oxygen to our red blood cells was one of those early metallic poisons. The hemoglobin molecule itself must have once, at the beginnings of cellular life, been formed to bind the newly dissolved atoms of metallic iron that entered the cell, to keep them from poisoning the cell itself. Today magnesium, also once poisonous, links together the important cellular enzymes that turn sugars into fuel. Calcium atoms speed impulses down our nerves.

But it is the neutralized, once-poisonous oxygen that serves us best. When life began there was no oxygen in the atmosphere; what little there might have been came from the interaction of the heated water vapor in the primitive atmosphere with the high-energy ultraviolet radiation flooding in from the sun. During the time when peptides and polymers were first appearing in the seas, and simple membranes were beginning to take a tentative hold on evolution, there was for all practical purposes nothing in the atmosphere but moisture. With no canopy of covering gases to absorb or deflect the beams of high-energy radiation that poured down from the sun onto the earth's surface, with no covering to protect the beginnings of life from those deadly cosmic gamma and beta rays, mutation followed mutation.

For over a billion years, the warm waters of the earth were churned and heated by those penetrating high-energy beams, driving the evolutionary process while at the same time killing it. So deadly must have been the surface of the early oceans that nothing could exist there. The membranes and polymers, the enzymes coming close to the surface would have been burned away, destroyed. Life had to evolve below the surface, at levels deeper than those cosmic rays would penetrate. It has been calculated from penetration studies of high-energy radiation that the first green cells had to develop at depths of ten and twelve feet below the oceans' surface, deep enough for the water to filter out most of the ultraviolet radiation but still close enough to the surface for the cells to use the few rays of visual light still getting through as energy to make their own sugars. Those first photosynthetic cells able to make their own food began to predominate. Ancestors of today's blue-green algae, those early sugar-making cells, became life's dominant form and gradually took over evolution. Growing by the trillions of billions, they soon filled the oceans. Oxygen, formed as a by-product of their photosynthesis, diffused into the water around them, building up in concentration until it began to emerge slowly out of the waters into the atmosphere.

At first there was barely a trace in the atmosphere, less than one part per million—oxygen levels that today we could barely pick up even with our most sophisticated gas sensors. As the photosynthetic cells continued to multiply, more oxygen diffused into the air. The concentration gradually increased; a million years after the atmospheric concentration was one part per million, it became two parts, then one half of one percent, then one percent. The photosynthetic cells continued to pour this new gas into the atmosphere. It began to filter out the sun's radiation, and life protected by this new canopy of oxygen gas moved slowly to the surface of the oceans. But the new gas was as poisonous to developing life as the earlier metals draining off the continents had been to the first cells, getting into them, as the metals had once done; diffusing through their cell walls; disrupting membranes, as those first atoms of iron and magnesium had; oxidizing proteins; changing the charge of their internal structures; disrupting everything so that suddenly nothing would work. The weaker cells died just as their weaker ancestors, unable to protect themselves from the iron and zinc atoms, had perished.

Even today oxygen can be just as poisonous, just as deadly. During the early nineteen-fifties, hundreds of newborn infants were blinded by it. We did it to them ourselves, with our own technology. Premature infants having trouble breathing had always been given additional oxygen, but until twenty-five years ago there had been no airtight incubators. With their development and use, prematures were suddenly discovered to be going blind, the retinas of their eyes destroyed by the growth of a strange fibrous tissue. Doctors proclaimed a brand-new disease, retrolental fibroplasia. They had no idea that what they were seeing in those blinded eyes was one of the oldest diseases on earth—oxygen poisoning.

From the beginning the doctors realized they were dealing with a very strange disease. The scientists who began to study it noted early that it occurred only to prematures born in developed, industrialized areas—Europe, the United States, Canada and South Africa. Physicians were puzzled; they checked blood levels for this and that, drugs the mothers might have taken, genetic defects, possible trauma, family history, the possibility of infectious diseases; they could find nothing. Finally someone asked the question, why now? And why only premies? And then, why only premies in developed countries?

The right questions finally brought the right, though startling answer: the only thing different about these blinded newborns was the incubators they were put into. All those blinded had been placed in the new airtight incubators available only in industrialized countries. The doctors found that these incubators had been introduced into popular use a few weeks before the first case of retrolental fibroplasia was reported. In the mini-world of those incubators, the newborn premature infant was forced to breathe air in which the oxygen levels had been raised from 40 to 60 percent higher than had ever been achieved before. That incubator, like the earth's early atmosphere, trapped the oxygen and concentrated it.

The effects of this increased oxygen concentration on the developing immature cells of a premature infant's retina was the same as on the early cells developing in the first seas. The premies' retinal cells were destroyed by the oxygen, just as those first early cells must have been destroyed. The difference between the incubator and the first seas was that the original developing cells were exposed slowly, almost excruciatingly slowly, over millions of years to ever increasing oxygen concentrations. Those cells had the time to learn how to bind the oxygen before it killed them all, just as they had discovered how to bind the earlier metallic atoms; the retinal cells of the prematures didn't. The early cells that had been able to neutralize the poisonous oxygen gas as it entered through their cell walls, survived. The premature's cells, unable to bind all the oxygen presented so quickly, in such high amounts, were poisoned; their internal machinery was oxidized and they died, and with them the child's sight.

In the process of binding and neutralizing oxygen, the primitive cells with the nonpoisonous oxygen now available within them learned to use the bound oxygen as an energy source. Protection had again led to utilization, and the evolutionary result was explosive. Before the availability of the neutralized oxygen as an energy source, cells had to rely on the chemical reduction of sugars and fats for the energy they needed to divide and multiply, to move and to grow. Those early energy sources were poor low-yield fuels, and so life was sluggish and slow, remaining single-cellular and impotent. But oxygen changed all that. Just as man's ability to move at great speeds in a car or to fly in a plane had to await the development of the high-horsepower, low-weight internal-combustion engine, the ability of cells to move swiftly, to develop high-output protein synthesis, to be able to contract quickly, to grow rapidly, had to await the availability of a high-yield, low-weight source of fuel. Oxygen was that fuel. But it also was something else. In the hundred million years following the increased rise of oxygen to over one percent of the atmosphere, life began to move to the ocean surface. The oxygen diffusing into the atmosphere not only fueled evolution but filtered out the deadly ultraviolet radiation.

When the oxygen neared an atmospheric content of 10 percent, the canopy of protection it afforded was great enough to allow the newly developed oxygen-breathing life to move out of the oceans onto the land. The Devonian era with its sudden emergence of abundant amphibious life is evidence of the protection afforded by the layer of oxygen, and later, ozone.

The body has always, throughout evolution, devoted as much of its defensive economy to the fighting of environmental poisons as it has to fighting other organisms, but in that battle of poisons it has always had the time to win. The metals that came off the forming continents did not do so all at once but gradually, over millions and millions of years, giving the cell a chance to develop defenses. It was the same with oxygen. Nothing, though, would have survived a billion tons of DDT dumped into its world within a decade. The supersonic aircraft, whose chemical exhaust may remove the layers of ozone from the atmosphere and let through the damaging ultraviolet radiation that once so brutally punished the earth, could yet again end evolution—and all of us and all we know with it.

OUR BODY will take care of us if given the slightest chance. It already has the best of nature within it and will survive if we will only let it, if we give it just half the chance it has given and continues to give each of us.

Not only has it neutralized past poisons for us, but more recent poisons, too. Many diseases we used to think of as being caused by the bacteria themselves are not; they are caused by poisons bacteria make. Our body knows the difference and has developed defenses not only against the bacteria but against their poisons as well.

During their own evolution, bacteria developed ever newer chemical means of ensuring their own survival, chemicals that allowed them to grow better, to spread more quickly through our bodies, even to fight off our own newly developed antibodies and complement. The streptococci make a protein called hyaluronidase which, diffusing out through its cell wall, destroys the cement holding together human tissues, enabling

the streptoccoci to spread rapidly and escape the body's defenses. Erysipelas, or streptococcal infections of the skin, are
more deadly than staph infections because the body cannot wall
off the strep as well. From a scratch, the whole face can become
infected within an hour, an arm red and painful within half a
day; a streptococcal-infected scratch of the foot, getting into the
lymphatics of the leg and moving up in a thin red line, reaches
the groin within hours. The women who died of puerpural fever
died because the strep organisms infecting their womb were
able to use hyaluronidase to spread quickly through the tissues
of their uterus and out into their bloodstream, eventually to
their heart, lungs and kidneys, before their bodies could even
begin to fight back. They had no time to make antibodies, no
time for the infection to be contained, for their white cells to
do their job. The hyaluronidase of the strep cut through the
walls of their uterus, allowing the organisms to escape and
spread. Even with that enzyme, though, the body can still in
most cases destroy the strep unless the infection is in an unusual
place, like the uterus, or the number of infecting organisms is
so overwhelming that the body just cannot handle them all.

Tetanus is one of those diseases not caused by the spread
of the bacillus itself but by the poison it makes. None of the
manifestations of tetanus—the lockjaw, the seizures, the air
hunger—are due to the tetanus bacteria destroying tissues,
causing disease, but are rather the results of a poison called
tetanospasmin, which the organism makes after it enters the
body. This poison is picked up by the circulation and carried
away from the bacteria to all parts of the body, affecting the cells
of the nervous system. Tetanus is a disease of wounds. In order
to grow, the tetanus bacillus must be in an area of low oxygen.
Dirty, decaying wounds, tissues with no blood supply and there-
for with low to no oxygen are not only the perfect place for it
to grow but the only place, as the deaths of millions of wounded
soldiers have shown.

Being a throwback to the earlier times of evolution, the
tetanus bacillus cannot survive in areas of high oxygen concentration. To protect itself from that oxygen, the tetanus organism
exists in two forms. One form is a spore—a small, heavily coated,
seedlike structure resistant to almost everything, including oxygen—which can exist in the soil for up to two or three years at

a time. These spores are found everywhere in the world. Studies have shown millions of them in microscopic samples of seemingly ordinary earth—in the dung of horses and cows, in sand, in dust, even in hay. A shrapnel fragment blasting up off the ground or a ricocheting bullet splattered with dirt is almost certain to carry tetanus spores with it into the wound. A saber slash at Waterloo, a mini-ball at Gettysburg, grenade fragments on Guadalcanal, bombs dropped over the Ardennes, claymores in Nam, all carried dirt into the wounds they caused, and with the dirt the spores of the tetanus organisms. The tissue surrounding the wound begins to die, cutting off the oxygen, and with decreasing oxygen the tetanus spores suddenly molt, turning into bacteria that begin to divide and multiply, producing the tetanospasmin.

The toxin that soon floods the wound diffuses out into the healthy surrounding tissues, where it is picked up by the bloodstream and carried throughout the body. The poison affects the body's nerves, getting into the brain cells and interfering with its functioning, poisoning the sympathetic nervous system and the spinal cord, acting for all the world exactly like the drug strychnine. There are seizures, muscular rigidity and tense, unrelenting pain. The neck becomes stiff, the muscles of the jaw and face lock shut; viselike contractions of the chest muscles and spasms of the back twist the body into grotesque shapes. The tetanus-infected wound keeps pumping the toxin into the bloodstream, the muscles of the throat gradually clamp shut, breathing becomes difficult or impossible, profuse sweating with temperatures of 105 or 106 degrees occur, cardiac arrhythmias, and in well over 50 percent of those infected, finally, mercifully, death.

Those who survived did so for one of several reasons: the wound was minor, so that the body quickly resupplied the damaged area with blood, bringing the tissue oxygen level back to normal and killing the dividing tetanus bacillus; the number of spores contaminating the wound was minimal or were themselves destroyed in the blast that caused the wound; the tetanus infection was far enough away from the central nervous system, or the surrounding blood supply was so poor that the body had time to manufacture antibodies against the foreign tetanospasmin, neutralizing the circulating poison before it could get to the nerves.

The body's immune system, caring only about the chemistry of the attacker and nothing else, responds to that different chemistry, alive or dead, chemical or microbial, exactly the same way, producing antibodies against a dangerous poison as quickly and as efficiently as it does against any other attacker. In the case of tetanus it makes antibodies that couple with the tetanus toxin, neutralizing it before it can get to the brain or spinal cord. The rest of the body's defenses—its white cells, macrophages and complement—go in and destroy the tetanus bacillus itself, stopping any further production of the toxin. But if the wounds are great, the spore contamination excessive, death from tetanus is a certainty.

Yet in World War II, with 2.5 million men in the U.S. Army wounded, for the first time since men had fought and been wounded not one died of tetanus. No one died from it because of immunization—using a vaccine made against bacterial poisons. The theory involved in making and using such antipoison vaccines is the same as for all the others. The tetanus organisms are grown, the toxin they produce collected, changed chemically by formaldehyde or heating so it can't cause disease but not enough to change its molecular antigenicity, and then injected into the body. The immune system, responding to the attenuated poison, makes antibodies that will be available if the person is ever wounded in the future and his wound infected with the tetanus bacillus.

The symptoms of diphtheria, too, are not caused by a bacillus but by the diphtheria toxin it produces. The shots given in infancy, in addition to pertussis antigens, contain not only the attenuated tetanus toxin but the attenuated diphtheria toxin as well, giving immunity from all three diseases. Three injections, eight weeks apart, a booster—and fears that have been a part of mankind since children first coughed and men fought are gone and should be gone forever, as should, with the use of the other vaccines, the fears of polio, and measles, mumps and rubella.

But all the effort and concern, all the wisdom and work of men like Pasteur, Jenner, Enders, Salk, Sabin and Robbins did not remove the tetanus spores from the earth, nor destroy the wild polio or measles virus. Their achievements do not keep the rubella virus from trying to infect pregnant women, or diphtheria out of the throat of infants. Every one of these plagues is still there, in the air around us, in the water we drink, in the food we eat, waiting to attack. Yet today millions ignore the ever present threat, foolishly refusing what is offered, what has been so gruelingly and bitterly won for us.

In May of 1970 six doctors from the Chicago Board of Health, Section of Infectious Disease, the Division of Pediatrics at St. Luke's Hospital, the Public Health Service and the National Communicable Disease Center reported in the *Illinois Medical Journal* an outbreak of diphtheria. Between December 1969 and February 1970, twenty-one cases were diagnosed and documented in the Chicago area. Two children died from the disease. Seven of these patients had never been immunized; two had received only one of the necessary three shots, and three had no idea whether they had been immunized or not. Those patients with the full three shots had only mild disease.

Similar recent outbreaks of diphtheria have been reported in Florida, Texas and Arizona. Outbreaks of measles and polio, too, have occurred.

Immunizations have finally given each of us the edge. There need be no more wailing by the bedside, no more cripples pulling themselves through life, no more brains destroyed by the cold chemical mindlessness of crystalline viruses. Yet in every city in this country, because parents neglect to immunize their children, because governments forget the past and ignore the future, because physicians refuse or neglect to practice preventive medicine, well over 70 percent of all children today between the ages of one and four have not been adequately immunized. One-half to one-third are susceptible to measles, over half to polio. We are dooming our own. The iron lungs will be back again, the hospitals filled once more with the retarded and the blind. There will again be gnashing of teeth and the terrible cry of "Why me?" "Why mine?"

13

Mistakes of Nature

IN 1965, in the largest amphitheater at Johns Hopkins University Hospital, Dr. Robert A. Good was ridiculed by the lecturer during Saturday morning grand rounds—to the glee of the assembled physicians—for trying "again" to prove that another disease, rheumatoid arthritis, was auto-immune, that it was caused by the patient's own antibodies attacking his own joints. It was the typical antagonism to new ideas, but more was involved than usual. What hung in the balance was a whole new concept of disease.

By the mid-sixties, antibodies had become the major interest in medical research; the newest medical discoveries were all based on immunology. The importance of antibodies and complement in fighting disease and in protecting the body had by then been proved beyond any reasonable doubt. Knowledge of precisely how they worked was being expanded in every major medical center in the country. The form and structure of antibodies, what complement was, where both were made, how they circulated, what forces moved them—all were part of the increasingly active investigations that were going on at the time, with the promise of prestige, money and position for those making the right discoveries.

And now, in the midst of all that work, it was being pro-posed that antibodies could themselves be dangerous. More-over, there were at the time perfectly acceptable theories of-fered by the professors at Hopkins as well as at other medical centers for many of the diseases which Good was now attribut-ing to antibodies and complement gone awry.

It had become obvious by 1965 that our immune system was one of the reasons, if not the major reason, for our survival as a species. In all the wonder and the excitement of the new immunologic discoveries and all the benefits promised by them, it was held that our antibodies, our granulocytes and macro-phages, our complement and properdin, were all responsible for our protection and continued existence. Now this new won-der, our immune system, was being put in doubt. Even today, those in the medical profession who have to deal with what have proved to be auto-immune diseases suffer from a certain embar-rassment when explaining such diseases to patients who suffer from them. There is a sense in every publication and in every lecture on auto-immune disease that there is something not quite right with the facts, that what is being talked about really shouldn't be happening.

After all, it is a fact that our race survives because of our immune system; in the long run it does carry us on. But that is only from the long view; if we look closer, if we just look around us, we are faced with terrible questions. Those Hopkins profes-sors who laughed at Good forgot that nature's concern is species survival, not individual existence; that nature will, when given the choice, sacrifice the one so that the all can continue. They looked only at the bright side of immunology. Their own humanity, their own fears and their own desires got in the way of seeing the truth, and so they were able to laugh.

By the late sixties it was known that there were many differ-ent kinds of arthritis: infectious arthritis caused by bacteria get-ting into the joint space, infecting it, destroying the articulating tissues, causing pain, swelling and pus; rheumatic fever with its tender, swollen elbows and knees; the osteoarthritis of aging where the weight-bearing joints—the hips and the knees—after fifty or sixty years of use, begin to degenerate and then simply give out; chronic rheumatoid arthritis affecting the hands and wrists; "Charcot's joint" caused by syphilis. Whatever the type of arthritis, they all caused the same things: pain, limitation of movement, and in most cases, crippling deformities.

There was and still is another kind of arthritis, one that has always been with us, which for the most part affects only children, and girls more often than boys. It looks like rheumatoid arthritis, acts like rheumatic arthritis, but plainly is neither. The larger joints of these children's bodies are the ones affected; their knees and elbows, and sometimes, though rarely, even their wrists, can become so swollen and tender that the child refuses to move; even the slightest touch brings tears. There was another difference about this childhood arthritis; within two years some of the children unaccountably were dead. Joint disease does not kill you, nor did it these children. They did not die from their arthritis but from a mysterious kind of kidney disease, one that seemed to progress, to get worse as their joints deteriorated.

No one could explain this murderous kidney disease, what caused it, any more than they could explain the reason for the arthritis. There was a third concern—many of these children also had a skin rash, a very strange, specific rash restricted solely to their faces, beginning below the eyes, spreading out over the cheeks, and finally dropping down to right above the mouth. The relationship between the rash, the arthritis and the kidney disease was noted but ignored, and the disease, because the overtly painful and swollen joints were the most obvious part of the children's complaints, was continually confused with rheumatic fever or rheumatoid arthritis and diagnosed as one or the other, depending on the bias of the examining physician.

In the early sixties, other associations with this triad of arthritis, kidney disease and facial rash had been made. The children were also found to be anemic, a very strange type of anemia, in which their circulating red cells were destroyed even as they were produced, destroyed in the children's own bloodstream by unknown factors. Pericarditis, or inflammation around the heart, was likewise observed, as were swollen gastrointestinal tracts. Some of these children had changes in personality too; a few were even reported to have overt seizures.

WITHOUT ANYONE being aware of it, the truth about this strange and complicated type of arthritis had begun to be unraveled in the previous decade. It started with the use of a new medical procedure, the kidney biopsy.

A biopsy is the surgical removal of a part of an organ—a very tiny bit of it—from the body; it is the doctor's way of knowing exactly what he is dealing with without having to do major operative procedures. The removed piece is stained and put under the microscope, where, by looking at the tiny stained sections, he can tell what is going on within the whole organ. We are all familiar with one type of biopsy, the one made to determine if a lump in a woman's breast is malignant. (The term "breast biopsy" is an exaggeration. Actually what is removed is a part of the breast, specifically a section of the mass that is of concern.) The mass in the woman's breast could be anything— a cyst, an infected abscess, a benign tumor, a scar, a bruise, normal tissue too near the surface, or cancer. Just to look at the mass or feel it is no help in determining what it is. Disease is a cellular process. It is only when we can look at the tissue under the microscope, see exactly what the mass is made of, that we have the unequivocal answer to whether it is caused by an infective process and so filled with granulocytes and macrophages, normal tissue, or cancerous cells. At times biopsies give frightening answers, but at least they are truthful ones.

A lump in the breast is easy to biopsy, since the breasts are on the surface of the body. It is not the same with the internal organs. Drinking barium or taking a barium enema may show a mass lining the wall of the stomach or obstructing the large bowel. A chest film can show a huge lesion in the lungs, or a physician can feel a lump in a patient's throat. But to biopsy any of these masses, just to get to them, would take a major operation. The chest would have to be opened to get at the mass in the lung; the neck operated on to get at the nodule; the abdomen would have to be explored, the intestines pushed aside, the stomach cut open, incised, the colon sectioned, to get at their masses. And if the mass or lump is not malignant, the patient cannot simply be sent home the next day. There is the risk to the anesthesia, to the operation itself, to postoperative recovery; there is the continuing, unending risk of wound infections.

The patient, if the mass proves benign, might suffer more from the attempt to biopsy the lump than from the disease itself, so biopsies of the major internal organs have never become routine procedures. But this didn't mean that physicians gave up trying to get a piece of what could be a malignant growth, wherever it was, that they did not continue to try to find ways to be sure of their diagnosis and perhaps save their patient's life. In the effort to explore more masses, to see exactly what they are, to see whether a radical cancer operation has to be performed, chemotherapy begun, to be able to comfort or inform the patient, to give a definitive tissue diagnosis, new techniques for biopsies have continually been sought.

In the case of the stomach, a long tube made of a special optical fiber that could be swallowed was devised so that the mass could be looked at right where it is. Proctoscopes were developed so the same thing could be done for the rectum and colon. For the kidney, because of its position directly under the muscles of the back on either side of the spine, a long razor-sharp needle was constructed. Today kidney biopsies are performed as routinely as breast biopsies; we know now when a kidney can be biopsied safely, and when not. Experience has taught us that people with high blood pressure, blood-clotting disorders, congenitally malformed kidneys, should not be biopsied. In 1949, however, when the first kidney biopsies were undertaken, none of this was known, and so disasters occurred. The technique used then was basically the same as the one used today. By taking an X-ray of the abdomen, the physicians were able to determine exactly where the kidneys were. The skin and muscles over one of the kidneys was numbed and then the long sharp hollow needle was pushed through the muscles of the back, and into the kidney itself.

The technique was appropriate, but the art had not yet been developed. To obtain a noninjurious kidney biopsy is not just a matter of pushing a five-inch needle into somebody's back and hoping for the best. It is the feeling of knowing when you are near the kidney itself, when and how to have the patient stop breathing as the needle is advanced so that it will not act like a knife and slash the kidney as it moves back and forth with his breathing. It is knowing how far to push in the needle so that it won't go through the kidney into the liver, stomach or small bowel, and how to control any bleeding that might occur. All this had to be learned before this important and potentially lifesaving diagnostic procedure could be performed and not

turned into a life-threatening act in which an emergency operation might become necessary, and death a distinct possiblity.

Through the past twenty years, the art of biopsying kidneys
has been developed to the point where the risk to the patient
is in most cases minimal, indeed almost nonexistent. But back
in 1949, no one really knew how to do it. Some of the first
patients bled and had to have their kidneys removed. Doctors
who were initially enthusiastic about the possibility of being
able to biopsy kidneys began to stay away from the procedure
and then finally, after a few deaths, refused to do them. But in
the early fifties one man, a pediatric kidney specialist, faced up
to a basic truth of medicine: if you want to understand a disease,
you have to go to the organ affected and you have to look at it.
Speculation has no place in medicine; not, that is, when you
don't have to speculate. After all, as he was later to say, the
kidneys were there, with nothing but a quarter-inch of skin and
a half-inch of muscle between them and the doctor. He decided
to try once again to do renal biopsies.

In the years between 1949 and 1952, a new kidney biopsy
needle had been developed, one that removed the kidney tissue
from the body without the suction that had been used earlier.
In 1952 Robert Vernier, a pediatrician at the University of Minnesota Medical School, did the first kidney biopsy on a child ever
performed in America. He was looking for the cause of an illness
called nephrotic syndrome, a unique kidney disease in which
vast amounts of blood proteins are lost in the urine, so much so
that the children affected swell up, sometimes gaining twenty,
thirty and forty pounds of water, and may eventually die. The
biopsy Vernier did was successful; there were no complications.
He did more on other children with nephrotic syndrome, but
much to his sadness found nothing unique in any of the biopsy
specimens. The tissues he had taken from the kidneys of these
swollen, ill children looked exactly the same as tissues taken
from normal children.

One year before Vernier's arrival at the University of Minnesota, the medical school had purchased its first electron microscope. Work had begun in the thirties on a microscope using
high-energy electron beams rather than visual light to enlarge
the objects being examined 200,000 to 300,000 times more than
could be achieved with the then best light microscope. The

electronic needs of World War II had stopped all development on the new microscope, but after the war, work had begun again and by the early fifties the first electron microscopes were put into general production. Instead of giving a blurred image of inner cellular structures, this new instrument with its electron beam gave a clear, precise enlargement of an object as small as a molecule, 400,000 times smaller than a human cell.

Vernier, finding nothing useful by looking at his kidney biopsy specimens with the light microscope, wondered if perhaps the changes he felt had to be present in the kidneys of these diseased children might not be visible down at the subcellular level. He was certain that there had to be something different in these diseased kidneys; he would not accept as a fact that there was not something there to be found.

At night, the only time he had free from his other duties, he learned electron microscopy. Every evening when his regular work was done—when his own patients had been taken care of, his student lectures had been composed, his journals read, and articles written—he would go over to the medical school's electron-microscope room and with the help of a technician learn the laborious techniques of electron-microscopic tissue mounting, the physics and electronics necessary to use the scope effectively, and then finally, how to run it himself. Today, a full professor of pediatrics, clinical and research director of the prestigious Cardiovascular Research Institute at the University of Minnesota, president of the Upper Midwest Kidney Foundation, attending physician to the pediatric wards of the University of Minnesota, as well as lecturer, teacher and healer, Vernier can still be seen in his office at one or two o'clock at night, working to find a few more answers to the ever new questions of kidney disease, trying as always to help a few more children.

Back in 1952, sustained by nothing more than the feeling he had that there must be something in those nephrotic kidneys, he found what he had suspected. Under the electron microscope he saw that there was a difference between the kidneys from his diseased patients and the biopsy specimens he had obtained from normal children thought to have kidney disease. It was a small change, a change too small to have been seen by the light microscope, but it was there on the electron scope. A small part of the surface of the cells lining the filtering part of the diseased kidneys was flattened out, distorted and mis-shaped. The cells necessary to keep the proteins out of the urine and in the blood were indeed abnormal.

A month later Vernier made what proved to be an even more important discovery. Trying to find why those cells had become misshapen, he began to biopsy every child with kidney disease, whatever the cause, not only those children who were losing large amounts of protein but also those with blood in their urine, or indeed with any kind of kidney failure.

Late one night, working at the electron microscope, he noticed in a biopsy specimen taken from a child who had recently been admitted with the symptoms of facial-rash arthritis, anemia and kidney disease, lumps of a strange material, considerable amounts of it, deposited in the filtering part of the child's failing kidneys. Vernier rechecked the biopsy specimens taken from people with kidney failure from other known causes—infections, hypertension, stones, interstitial nephritis, poisons—but in none did he find the material that was so abundantly prevalent in the kidney-biopsy specimen of this child.

Over the next few months he did biopsies on other children admitted with these same bizarre and unexplained symptoms. To his great surprise and even greater excitement he found the same lumps of discrete material in all their kidneys. He rechecked all the biopsy specimens available to him, not only from those children admitted to the University of Minnesota but from other centers as well. He found this particular abnormality, those strange lumps of material, only in the children who were sick with the confusing multiple-system disease. The lumps, he proved, were not part of the kidney itself; they were abnormal deposits. Could they be the cause of the kidney disease? he wondered. But if so, what were they?

Vernier knew that before you can understand a disease, much less find a cure, you have to determine the cause. Perhaps with these children the deposits were part of the cause—and if they were, he reasoned, they should be in their other diseased organs as well—in their joints and skin. The great question was first to find out what this material was, and for that Vernier had help. The early fifties had been a time of great advancement in protein chemistry. Antibodies, known to be proteins themselves, were discovered circulating as gamma globulins in the bloodstream. At the same time, basic protein scientists had begun to use techniques to isolate, separate and purify these gamma globulins. Their methods were available to him.

At the same time other clinical specialists working in their own particular fields were also, like Vernier, caring for these multiple-system afflicted children. Some of these children, suffering more from their anemia than from their kidney disease, were being cared for by hematologists. Others, with their terrible facial rash, had been sent to dermatologists. Many, because of the problem of their joints, were being seen by rheumatologists. The popular notion of the medical researcher working in isolation, of one dedicated man following a medical or surgical idea through from beginning to end all by himself, no longer holds true; it is not a part of today's medicine. Modern methods of communication are too extensive, the distribution of information too instantaneous and widespread for any one man to do or be allowed to do the whole thing himself—if, that is, others find his ideas or observations relevant or potentially worthwhile.

The publication of an important observation or the introductory data to a new idea or theory is quickly circulated through the whole medical world. A medical research lab in La Jolla, California, begins to gear up to look at the blood of patients with a disease similar to one described just days before in an article published in an English medical journal. A clinician in New York changes the dosages of an experimental drug because of a recent case report from Canada's Toronto Children's Hospital. It is this rapid interchange of ideas that in recent years has led to the astonishing growth in our understanding of the physical aspects of disease. It was critical to our unraveling the reason for the suffering in these children with the triad of arthritis, anemia and kidney failure, critical for our understanding the disease that was eventually to be called by the ponderous name systemic lupus erythematosus.

In the late forties a hematologist at the Mayo Clinic, attending patients suffering from a strange type of iron-resistant, unexplained and unexplainable anemia, found during routine examination of their blood smears something he had never seen before in any person's circulation, healthy or diseased—a strange, bizarrely staining new kind of blood cell. There were not many of these cells. He had to look at hundreds of blood smears from the same person before he saw even one, but they were there in every patient with this kind of anemia. Sooner or later, if he did enough smears he would find at least one of these muddy-red–colored cells among the patient's normal, brightly stained red and white cells. They were the only thing he found that all these anemic patients had in common. But common findings in an uncommon disease gives the researcher a place to begin, a cue to pursue.

Surprisingly, when these bizarre cells were examined, they appeared to be nothing more than white cells that had eaten lumps of some kind of strange amorphous material. Any hematologist has during his years of experience seen blood smears showing white cells in the process of eating, or rather engulfing, bacteria. These strange new cells—eventually called LE cells for the disease of which they were to become so much a part (lupus erythematosus)—looked for all the world just like white cells that had eaten something, only the material engulfed was certainly not a bacterium.

What was it? Working seventy miles apart, hematologist and kidney specialist were faced with the same problem. The answer came slowly. It was the hematologists who led the way. In an attempt to identify what the material in the LE cell was, or at least where it came from, they took serum from patients with these strange cells in their bloodstream and white cells from normal people, and incubated the two together. They were trying to find out by this simple experiment whether the substance engulfed by the white cells, turning them into the circulating LE cells, was something in the serum of these anemic patients.

In scientific terms, it was a long assumption, a rather far-out idea, but it proved productive. The same cells that had been seen in the blood smears of the anemia patients were formed right there in front of the researchers in the test tube. Obviously the engulfed material, whatever it was, was circulating in the blood of these anemic patients. Other hematologists read the reports and began experiments of their own.

Reading the published reports of experimental work being done with the blood of these anemic patients, Vernier found mention of the fact that besides having the strange LE cells in their circulation, the patients also had blood and protein in their urine. It was no more than a sentence or two in each report, but it was enough for Vernier to realize that some of these patients, seen only by hematologists, must also have had unrecognized kidney disease, and that the substance engulfed by their white cells might also be the same kind of material he had found in the diseased kidneys of his own ill and anemic children.

The kidney receives 1,440 liters of blood a day. Any material in the blood, even in small amounts, could readily accumulate in the kidney, each liter of blood depositing a small but continuing amount of this substance, so that over a period of time a large amount would build up, enough so that by using the light microscope, he would be able to see it as deposits in his biopsy specimens. Perhaps the blood was the origin of these kidney deposits.

Since Vernier was an expert in the microscopic study of tissues, he knew that one of the ways to test his new theory and try to identify the material in the kidneys was to stain his biopsy tissue with specific chemical dyes, and see which of the stains the strange substance took up.

From the beginnings of microscopy, histologists, as a way of trying to identify cellular elements, have been developing ever more specific chemicals which, because of their own molecular properties, would stick to and color individual structural elements of cells and tissues. Some dyes stain only cellular connecting fibers, others only proteins, a few only cell nuclei, others only cytoplasm. Some dyes are specific for fats, and still others only for sugars and proteins; one or two can even be used to pick out specific subcellular enzymes.

Vernier stained each microscopic biopsy section with every dye available, but the lumps of material did not stain well with anything. They took up a little of the stain for materials containing a bit of sugar, but no more. Perhaps the material was covered with something that kept the right dye from really taking. Perhaps it was made up of different kinds of substances, none in sufficient quantity to stain heavily enough with any one dye to be identified. Perhaps the fixation of the tissue or the sectioning process had so changed the material itself that it was simply not the same as in its natural state, and therefore unstainable.

Vernier would never have found an answer if histological research had stopped with the development of only chemical stains. If you want to identify specific chemical materials you must, as with people, be able to pick out more than just the general characteristics, more than the fact that the person has two legs, two arms and a head. You must be able to notice the unique specific features of that person, the way his nose is shaped, the special configuration of his jaw and chin.

At the time that Vernier was trying with no success to identify the material in his kidney specimens, using chemical dyes that despite their sensitivity were still specific only for general classes of compounds, one of his young associates, Alfred Michael, another pediatrician at the medical school, was using a newly developed staining technique that not only could identify the presence of minute amounts of proteins in tissues, but could tell if those proteins were antibodies and, if antibodies, which kind—IgA, IgG or IgM. Michael's technique could also be used to specifically pick out complement and properdin.

With Michael's help, Vernier overlayed the biopsy specimens with the new immunofluorescent stain. To their surprise they found that the lumps of material in these diseased kidneys were proteins, and more startling, that the proteins were IgG antibodies. They used the same immunofluorescent staining techniques on the material inside the LE cells which they had found in a few of their kidney patients' blood smears. They found that this, too, was antibody.

These were discomforting discoveries. The material in the LE cells and the deposits of material in the diseased kidneys were both antibodies, and more important, the same type of antibody. Vernier and Michael knew that antibodies don't just circulate in the bloodstream. They are made against some attacker, some foreign substances. They also knew that white cells just don't go around eating up things. They will begin to engulf particles only if those particles are first coated with antibodies, and the only particles they knew of that could be covered with antibodies were bacteria. But none of these patients were infected.

Vernier and Michael discussed their new discoveries with Good, who even then at his young age was already a full professor at Minnesota.

Two big questions were quickly raised, questions with gigantic consequences for both patients and medicine, questions that had never been asked before. The three men knew they were out alone at the borders of medical science. It seemed to them that the antibodies they had found in the children's kidneys and in the LE cells found in a few of their bloodstreams had to be involved in some way with their disease. They were not the least bit comfortable or even willing to say that the cause of the kidney disease and the anemia were these antibodies, but they were equally as sure that they were somehow related. After all, Vernier had not found the deposits of antibody anywhere except in diseased kidneys, never in normal ones, and the hematologists had not described one single LE cell in anyone without the iron-resistant anemia. Moreover, others had reported the presence of LE cells circulating in the blood of children with joint disease as their main complaint, their rash, anemia and kidney disease being secondary.

The three physicians reviewed the possibilities of what had been found, and despite their own reluctance, came back again and again to the same seemingly impossible position—the involvement of the antibodies themselves in the disease. After months of looking they still had not found a single instance of antibody deposits in a kidney biopsied from a normal person, nor in the serum of a healthy child or adult. Each night the three went home a bit more uncomfortable, a bit more uneasy about their conclusion.

IT MAY SEEM a long way from LE cells and human kidney disease to the New Zealand white rabbit—until we remember that the rabbit, too, had its beginnings with us in those primeval seas, that its battles have been our battles, its methods of defense our methods, its immune mistakes our own. It was these rabbits that gave the three researchers the proof they needed to show that antibodies could be dangerous, that they were indeed the cause of the rash, the anemia, the arthritis and the deadly kidney disease called systemic lupus erythematosus.

The proof began with Good's realization that these same symptoms had been seen before by physicians, had in fact occurred decades earlier in almost epidemic proportions.

There was a time in the late twenties and thirties, before the discovery of antibiotics, when in the desperate attempt to halt the spread of gangrene, to try to save children with meningitis, to cure pneumonia, patients were injected with foreign substances; indeed, such injections had become a national event. The work of Pasteur, Metchnikoff, Durham, Ehrlich, the immunologic insights of Bordet, Fleming, Zinsser and Webb, had by that time finally been accepted by the medical profession and brought into general therapeutic use in an attempt to treat infections.

It is difficult for us today to realize the desperation of yesterday's physicians having to treat pneumonias by sitting helplessly by the bedside waiting for the fever to break so they could then tell the family everything would be all right. It is hard for us to remember how fatal meningitis was, how physicians could do nothing but stand there and watch their patients die. But with the proven successes of vaccinations, the development of standardized antitoxins, Bordet's elucidation of the action of complement and antibody on bacterial destruction, the explanation of the differences between immediate and delayed hypersensitivity, the discovery of antibacterial antibodies in serum, procedures for purifying antibodies, and the precise methods for determining their types and amounts—physicians with no place else to go, finally turned in the early decades of the twentieth century to the only science available with any theory to deal with the infections that were killing their patients: the new science of immunology.

Anything was better than doing nothing, and the new immunologic understanding and techniques at least made scientific sense, so the methods that had been used in the laboratory began to be used on people. An antibody industry developed in this country that rivaled today's pharmaceutical empires. The ideas that enabled it to happen were all immunologically sound, theoretically correct and by the late thirties technically possible. Pure cultures of disease-causing bacteria—the meningococcus that causes meningitis, the pneumonococcus that causes pneumonias, the streptococcus that causes scarlet fever—were injected into large animals—for convenience, horses—so that large amounts of blood could later be withdrawn. A few days after the inoculation the animals were bled, their serum collected and the antibodies concentrated. The concentrated serum containing antibodies against the human disease-causing bacteria were then used as treatment, injected back into people in the hopes that it would help them fight their infection. In simple terms, what the physicians were trying to do was give preformed antibodies to already infected people. Yet so new were the theories of immunology—in truth, so little was known then about how our immune system really works—that the treatments were never really effective; in many cases the injections themselves proved potentially life-threatening. Yet with terrible bacterial infections a constant everyday occurrence, the horse-serum industry grew.

All over this country, and indeed, all over the world, serum from horses that had been infected with human disease-causing bacteria were injected into people's veins. Patients with meningitis or pneumonia, typhoid fever or diphtheria, scarlet fever or gangrene, were given injections. Children suffering from osteomylitis, soldiers dying from pus-filled wound infections, all were treated the same. In truth, horse-serum injections were becoming, like antibiotics today, an expected part of medical treatment, when literally overnight the discovery of penicillin and streptomycin put an end to it.

Within months of the discovery of antibiotics, the great horse-serum industry virtually disappeared. The industry's stocks became worthless, and thousands of workers, manufacturers and distributors were forced to find other jobs. Buildings and barns were sold. Inside of a year no signs remained of what had fast become the largest health-care industry in this country. The serum industry collapsed so quickly not only because antibiotics were more effective—in medicine, two or three forms of therapy often continue to exist side by side—but because the horse serum injections had proved dangerous. Many patients given these injections began, after a few treatments, to develop a strange new disease—a disease called, appropriately, serum sickness.

In the first few months after injections with horse serum had begun, it was noticed that some people receiving a second injection, even if they recovered from their infection, went on within two weeks of the second treatment to develop fever, to have joint pains; a few began to show blood and protein in their urine; some even had skin rashes. A third injection could kill the patient, and a number did die. When the patients who had died were autopsied, it was found that the blood vessels throughout

[177]

their bodies were inflamed, swollen, broken open, oozing, as if the person had taken some kind of caustic poison. Those with kidney disease were found to have lumps of an undiagnosable material deposited throughout their kidney tissues.

Serum sickness had continued to puzzle physicians long after the serum industry had ceased to exist. Unexplained, it remained a source of interest and concern to a number of medical researchers. Good, who knew of the problem and had once reviewed all the original case reports pertaining to serum sickness, suddenly realized the similarity of symptoms between these patients and the children with lupus. He began his own experiments.

Horses were too big to handle, so he turned to laboratory animals—New Zealand white rabbits. The question was to find out what it was in the horse serum that caused disease in the patients with serum sickness. Perhaps it would shed some light on what was wrong with the children with lupus.

Good started, as had others who were studying serum sickness, as simply as he could; he injected his experimental rabbits with horse serum. With the second injection the rabbits acquired a disease exactly the same as serum sickness in man. Since cows were more easily available than horses, he tried cow serum, and again with the second injection the rabbits began to suffer from arthritis, fever, kidney disease and rash.

Work on experimental serum sickness was also going on in other medical centers. Researchers finding what Good had found proceeded to the next logical step: they fractioned the cow's blood into its components—sugars, fats, carbohydrates and proteins. Injecting each pure fraction, they found that it was on the second injection of only the protein fractionated of the cow's blood that the disease occurred. The disease in the injected rabbits was exactly the same as in the serum sickness in humans. It had the same time course as human serum sickness, the same organ involvement, the same vessel inflammation, the same kidney deposits. Indeed, as with people, a third injection of the cow protein would also kill some of the rabbits.

The deposits that were found in the rabbits' diseased kidneys were found to be antibodies, but even more important, deposits of the same antibodies were found wherever there was any vascular inflammation.

It was obvious that the rabbits had made antibodies against the injected cow protein, which their immune system had read as foreign. Perhaps the same thing had happened in humans when they'd been injected with horse serum. In that serum, as Good knew, mixed in with other horse proteins were the antibodies that were the whole reason for the injections. Perhaps the humans with serum sickness had made antibodies against the injected horse proteins. Theoretically it could happen. But how and why did this cause disease?

Work with the rabbits continued and the story began to unfold. The first injection of the cow protein caused the production of antibodies by the rabbits' immune system. When the rabbits' blood was removed and examined after the first injection, it was found that most of the rabbits had a marked increase in circulating antibodies specific for cow protein. Within hours after the second injection, a gigantic increase in antibody levels occurred in these same rabbits, and with that increase, the beginnings of disease.

The injected rabbits were sacrificed one, two, three, four, five and six days after they had received the second injection of foreign protein. On the second day, even before the rabbits had become overtly ill, their small blood vessels, mysteriously coated with what once had to be circulating antibodies, were undergoing injury; the cells lining the arteries, capillaries and veins were found on examination under the microscope to be beginning to degenerate. By the fourth day after the injection, granulocytes and lymphocytes had moved into the diseased areas and begun eating their own antibody-coated cells as if the coated vessel wall cells were foreign invaders. Day by day, as the rabbits' immune response increased, as more antibodies, complement, granulocytes and macrophages entered the already diseased areas, the tissue injury became worse and the animals looked sicker. A third injection caused a terrifying bodily reaction: almost instantaneously the animals' lungs filled with fluid, their vessels that were inflamed broke open and bled, their hearts dilated, their kidneys turned white, and within minutes the animals were dead.

But the medical establishment still found it hard to accept the idea of antibodies causing disease. After all, not every human given injections of horse serum acquired serum sickness, and not every rabbit given cow protein became ill.

The confusion arising with the rabbit studies, which kept Good and his fellow researchers from definitively saying that antibodies could cause disease, was that not all the rabbits being injected with the foreign protein responded in the same way. Hundreds of rabbits were used, all injected with the same amount of cow protein, yet some did not develop disease. It was discovered later the animals that were spared were the ones whose immune systems for some reason failed to produce great amounts of antibody against the injected material. A second group produced slightly higher levels of antibody and they had some mild kidney disease but did not become too ill, even after a third or fourth injection. The third group, which developed high levels of antibodies, were the ones that had the full-blown disease. They were the sickest, the ones with the arthritis, the terrible kidney disease, the vessel disease and the rash, and they were the ones that died after a third injection.

Those opposed to the idea that antibodies could be harmful seized on this seeming confusion, much as today's physicians who refuse to accept cigarette smoking as a cause of lung cancer, or preservatives as a possible cause of cancer, seize on the statistical nature of those studies to try to prove their points. And of course, as the detractors pointed out, one great question still existed. How did the antibodies cause the tissue injury to the rabbits' own cells? The work continued, and after ten years of constant effort, of one experiment after another, the answer was found.

By the late sixties it had been proved beyond any doubt that the disease of serum sickness in man and in the rabbit was caused by the production of antibodies against the injected foreign proteins. In the case of humans, their immune system read the horse protein injected into their bodies as foreign; with the rabbits, it was the cow protein.

It was discovered that the rabbit's antibodies combined with the antigens on the cow's foreign proteins, and the protein-antibody complexes circulating in the rabbit's bloodstream got stuck as they traveled through the animal's body in the small blood vessels of the joints, heart, lungs and kidneys, and once there, activated any passing complement, causing injury to the cells or to the tissues on which they happened to settle out. It was that simple; foreign substances were injected directly into the bloodstream. Antibodies were made against them that combined with them; these antigen-antibody complexes continued to circulate until in their circuit through the body they entered the tiny vessels where they got caught; and once caught, activating complement, blew holes in the vascular cells they got stuck on—injuring the vessels and eventually the organs in which those vessels were located.

Serum sickness, it was realized, was a disease of chance. If the circulating antigen-antibody complexes—and in the high antibody producers there were billions—got stuck in the kidneys, the human or rabbit acquired kidney disease. If the complexes were deposited in the joints, there was joint disease; in the skin, skin rashes. If they were deposited all over, there was death.

Serum sickness was the first documented example of disease being caused by the immune system's mistakenly reading injected harmless proteins as potentially dangerous foreign invaders and going after them with the same blindness and ruthlessness with which it attacks its real enemies—the poisons, viruses and bacteria.

14

The Body
Against Itself

THE FIRST STUDIES on serum sickness pointed the way toward a new kind of thinking about disease, that antibodies could be harmful; perhaps not intentionally harmful, but that made little difference to the people suffering from those diseases, who were crippled or killed because of their own antibodies. But the children with lupus whose joints and kidneys were being ruined, and the anemic adult patients with the LE cells in their serum, had never been exposed to any foreign material, had never been given an injection of any foreign protein. If Good was right and the patients with lupus, like the humans with serum sickness and rabbits injected with foreign proteins, were suffering from a disease caused by antibody production, then what were those antibodies made against?

For years no one knew. One dead end followed another. Then in the late sixties a tiny little animal, the Aleutian mink, provided the answer—and with it, a whole new understanding of human disease.

IN EARLY 1941, on an Oregon mink ranch, a deadly mutation had occurred in the course of a mink-breeding experiment. Almost overnight a large number of the expensive newborn minks were found dead in their cages. With the possibility of an infectious epidemic, veterinarians were called in. The dead animals were autopsied and it was discovered that their vessels were inflamed, their kidneys injured, their joints and hearts and skin damaged. But no microbes were found. The autopsy findings were collected and published in the *Journal of Natural Fur News* under the title "Aleutian Mink Disease."

Because of the deaths, the breeding experiments were stopped and there were no further cases. But the disease continued to arise spontaneously at intervals over the years. When it occurred again in the sixties, new articles were published. By this time, medical researchers involved in the study of antibody disease were scanning the world's literature for any clues to the possible causes of antibody production, and seeing these articles, realized what they had found: a new animal model of a serum sickness–like disease where there had been no injections, a truly naturally occurring disease like that found in patients suffering from lupus.

Minks were purchased for medical research and experimentally bred to cause the disease; similar genetic types, but without the disease, were used as controls. Serum, bone marrow, lymph nodes, livers, hearts, kidneys of newborn diseased and normal animals were studied. The microscopic sections of the diseased tissue from the affected animals all showed lumps of material in them—antibody—as well as white cells and complement. The closeness of these findings to those in the vessels and organs of the rabbits, in humans with serum sickness, and children with lupus, was obvious. But what had caused the production of those antibodies?

A paper published in the *Proceedings of the Society of Experimental and Biological Medicine* gave part of the answer. Heyman, a researcher at Yale, described a series of his own experiments which, had they been generally known, not only would have stopped those Hopkins professors from ridiculing Good and his ideas of antibodies causing disease but would have made the discussion of auto-immune diseases—of our immune system making antibodies against our own tissues—the major topic in every medical school in the world.

What Heyman did was take the kidneys out of young healthy rats, grind them up and inject these minced kidneys into other rats of the same species. Within days the injected rats began to have blood and protein in their urine; a few more days and it was obvious they all had begun to develop severe kidney disease. When the animals' diseased kidneys were examined, huge amounts of antibody were found in them, right in the areas of worst damage; large amounts of complement were also found along with the deposits of antibody.

The importance of these experiments centered on the fact that there was absolutely nothing unique about the kidneys that Heyman had ground up to inject. They were all healthy, sterile and exactly the same structurally, morphologically, chemically and biologically as the kidneys of the injected rats. Yet the injection of similar tissues, exactly like their own, had plainly induced the immune system of the injected rats to make antibodies against them. Injected with normal tissues exactly like their own, these injected animals had somehow misread those tissues as foreign. Not only that, but the antibodies had ended up back in their kidneys, causing terrible injury.

Injected only with kidney tissue, these animals had made antibodies specific to kidney cells; antibodies made against the ground-up kidneys had gone on to attack their own. Clearly, the kidneys that Heyman removed had had their surfaces changed enough in the removal or had had new antigens exposed in the grinding to be read as foreign when injected into the healthy rats. Antibodies had been made against these "foreign" cells, but their surfaces, even changed, were still so close to the surfaces of the injected rats' normal kidneys that the antibodies they produced cross-reacted with their own kidneys, going after them, too, and causing disease.

Heyman's studies showed that antibodies could be made specifically against an animal's own tissues, that we could indeed make antibodies against ourselves. But he had injected ground-up kidneys to prove the point. The Aleutian mink showed that it could happen naturally.

For years, researchers had tried to discover why. In 1968, using new viral techniques, they found that all the diseased minks were infected with a virus. The new theory, based on

Heyman's work and the Aleutian mink discoveries, was unclut-tered and simple. It was proposed that Aleutian mink disease was caused by antibodies produced against an infecting virus. With the mutation occurring spontaneously or during breeding, a chemical or biological change took place in the mutated minks' immune system that allowed the virus, perhaps present in the bodies of all minks but normally kept in check, to sud-denly grow. Becoming infected, these mutated minks began to make antibodies against the infecting virus now spreading through their bodies. It was then the same thing that had hap-pened to humans with serum sickness and the rabbits injected with cow protein. The circulating antigen-antibody complexes that developed got stuck in the animals' smaller vessels and caused injuries.

It was also theorized, based on Heyman's work, that the infecting virus, having gotten into the minks' cells, changed some of those infected cells so that they were read as foreign, and antibodies were made against them that cross-reacted with all the still-healthy cells in the minks' bodies, causing continu-ally more widespread disease. A chain reaction was proposed: a few infected cells caused a small anticellular antibody produc-tion; these antibodies also attacked normal cells which pro-duced more damaged cells, and those in turn caused more an-tibodies that went after still more normal cells which caused still more antibodies to be produced, using up more and more com-plement, bringing in more and more granulocytes, macro-phages and lymphocytes into the diseased areas, causing ever more disease.

These experiments and observations led to more observa-tions, all strengthening the concept of auto-immune disease. Within years of Heyman's work and the discovery of the viral, antibody cause of Aleutian mink disease, it was also found ex-perimentally that naturally occurring thyroid hormone—itself a protein—when slightly altered chemically and injected into the very animal it had been removed from, caused anti-thyroid antibody production that would attack the animal's own thyroid gland, causing thyroiditis, or inflammation of the gland. The antibody the animal's immune system had made against the altered hormone also cross-reacted and went after not only the normal hormone itself but even the gland that produced it.

THE PROOF of any medical theory ultimately lies in its application to human disease. All the definitive proofs of auto-immunity thus far had come only from experimental work, from animal studies or from humans under the artificial conditions of being injected with altered or foreign proteins. The medical world, still skeptical, waited for the first proof that antibodies could naturally cause disease. That first proof came finally through the understanding of a specific type of thyroid disease.

Pediatric endocrinologists had always been faced with the problem of the once bright child, formerly so alert and active, who is brought sullen, lethargic, into their office. Sleepy, sluggish, twenty pounds overweight, not able to or not caring to respond to anything, the child sits on the examining table, the face unemotional, masklike, while the frightened and worried parents give a history of a week or two of fever, generalized lethargy, a tender, swollen neck and then over the next few weeks or even months a gradual downhill course from the happy, lively child they knew to this sullen, lifeless, apathetic patient.

And the child is indeed lifeless; his heart rate is slow, even his reflexes are diminished. His skin, thick and doughy, has none of the smoothness and elasticity of childhood or adolescence. The thyroid gland in his neck is small and rock-hard; in a few children it might still be even a bit tender.

It had been known for years that these children had thyroid disease, and this was attributed to infected thyroid glands. It was startling to find, when their diseased glands first began to be biopsied, that they were not filled with infection but instead looked exactly like the diseased glands of the experimental animals which were injected with their own altered thyroid hormone. They were filled with the same deposits of antibody, the same hordes of lymphocytes as the thyroids of the experimental animals. There could be only one explanation for the similarity in the thyroid pictures. These children, too, had to be making auto-antibodies against their own thyroid hormone. And that was the case: the children were found to have anti-thyroid antibodies in their circulation which would couple with thyroid hormone.

Somehow these children's hormone, either in production

or distribution, had been altered while it was still in their bodies, and this alteration, causing a change in the hormone's protein structure, perhaps even as little a change in its structure as one or two amino acids, was enough to be read by their ever vigilant immune system as foreign, read by a billion years of chemical evolution as the enemy, as different, no longer as "self," and so attacked, hunted down, followed even into the gland where the hormone itself was made. The immune system was trying to stop the production of the altered hormone—to save the body from a nonexistent threat as if the gland were producing bacteria instead of hormone—trying to kill the source of the altered hormone, to stop its spread by keeping it from being formed, and in the process destroying any still-normal hormone as well as the gland itself.

The lethargy, the heart failure, and the mental slowness and apathy of these thyroid-deficient children were all caused by the fanatic within them, a fanatic that in its blind effort to protect their bodies will go on to destroy what it has been trained to protect, the children themselves.

THE FINAL unequivocal proof that antibodies can and do cause disease, the proof that would silence skeptical physicians forever, was found in those very children who years before had caused the whole search to begin—Vernier's children with the triad of rashes, arthritis and kidney disease. Vernier, Michael and Good already knew that these children had antibodies in their diseased kidneys. The hematologists had proved that the LE cell was made up of antibodies eaten by white cells. The dermatologists had discovered both antibodies and complement in the skin of these patients in the areas of their rashes. Other researchers had found antibodies and complement in the small vessels of those lupus patients with vascular and joint disease.

But the question still remained: What was the specificity of the antibody in lupus? What was it made against? It wasn't made against an altered protein or cell or a microbe or any kind of injected material. The researchers kept searching; more delicate, more specific ways of looking for antibodies were developed. Eventually, using these new methods, it was established that the antibodies in these patients' serum reacted unexpectedly, in fact coupled with the nucleus of their own cells, specifically their DNA, the basis of life.

Hidden inside the nucleus of our cells, the DNA is separated from the outside world of all our blood and tissue fluids— by the nuclear membrane, the cell's cytoplasm, and outside of the cell itself, its surrounding plasma membrane. Somehow, in those patients suffering from lupus erythematosus, the DNA gets out of a few of the cells and into the bloodstream, where it had never been before. Once there, it is read by the patient's immune system as a foreign substance, and antibodies are manufactured to attack it. Like a sentry familiar with every chemical constituent of the body, the immune system is suddenly faced with a large, unfamiliar molecule which is and has always been a part of the body but which, hidden away inside the cells, has never before been presented to the immune system. And so, in its own unrestricted confidence, the immune system goes after the DNA as it would any foreigner.

In the early seventies, using immunofluorescent-labeling techniques, researchers were able to locate the DNA itself sitting in the diseased areas of the kidneys of these children with lupus, coupled to their anti-DNA antibodies, proving beyond question that the disease was the result of these patients' making antibodies against normal parts of their own bodies, that it was indeed auto-immune.

But again, why the antibody production? We know that physical agents such as the ultraviolet radiation of sunlight can destroy skin cells, causing the release of the DNA from their nuclei into the bloodstream. Then, too, cellular injury, such as from viral infections, may release nuclear DNA into the bloodstream. It was also possible that the patient with lupus might be making antibodies directly against the infecting viral DNA itself. Perhaps, like the Aleutian mink, the lupus patients are born with a genetic defect which makes them susceptible to a DNA virus the rest of us can resist. Whatever, these patients make anti-DNA auto-antibodies, which combine with the free DNA in their circulation, and like the antigen-antibody complexes of the people with serum sickness, the complexes get deposited out in their organs, causing tissue injury and disease.

We have come a long way, but patients still suffer from lupus. At a recent conference Vernier and Michael, both now full professors of pediatrics and universally acknowledged experts on the disease, felt compelled to warn a new group of pediatric interns that although we know a good deal about the mechanisms involved in lupus, it is still a lifelong disease and patients still die from it.

AUTO-IMMUNE DISEASE has become a concept no one can any longer ignore. Rheumatic fever, for instance, is now known to be such a disease. It is caused by a streptococcal infection of the throat, but the rheumatic-fever part of the disease—the joint involvement, the rash and valvular heart disease—is the result of an immune response being mounted against the strep in the throat. The T and B cells produced for some reason mistake the child's heart muscle and joints for the attacking streptococci and go after them with the same determination that they go after the strep in his throat. The infectious-disease experts feel that there is some antigenic similarity that goes way back in evolution between heart muscle, joint tissues and the streptococcus organism itself, at least enough similarity so that the antibodies made against the streptococcal surfaces become confused and attack the cell membranes of their own body, damaging joints and hearts, causing crippling heart failure and at times death.

Hay fever, too, is an auto-immune disease. As in a patient with serum sickness, the tissues of the allergic patient are injured as innocent bystanders. They are damaged because they are near the destructive chemical reaction of the immune response.

If hay fever is not as deadly an immune complex disease as lupus or serum sickness, it is because the immune reactions that occur in the hay-fever patient are restricted to the surface of his body, not to deeper, important organs. In this disease the antigen is not a foreign circulating protein—neither a virus, nor DNA—but pollen grains, some less than six microns in diameter, smaller than a living cell, some even smaller than bacteria. These golden grains, too tiny to be seen, get into the covering of our eyes, the mucous membranes of our nose and even, because of their small size, past the sticky secretions of our trachea and down into the very lining of our bronchus.

Our immune system goes after these pollen grains as if they

were alive. But since they are not, they can't be killed, nor at the same time can they move any farther down into our body. They just stay on the surfaces, where the body blindly throws more and more IgA antibodies, more and more complement, more and more lymphocytes at them—like an army wasting its rockets against uncaring boulders. The whole surrounding area containing the pollen grains—the bronchus, the lining of the eyes, the mucous membranes of our nose—becomes the battlefield; the chemical mediators—histamine, serotonin—released by the antibody reaction, and complement as well, pulverize the normal tissues on which the pollen grains sit. They remain while the cells around them are caught up and injured by the chemical mediators, becoming swollen and reddened and keeping us miserable, unable to breathe or to see normally. We cough, our eyes itch, and our nose runs; we wheeze and feel terrible.

The antihistamines, the epinephrine, the mist sprays that doctors prescribe to relieve the misery of hay fever have nothing to do with the removal of the pollen grains, nor with stopping our antibodies from coupling with them; all they do—and in most cases it is enough—is interfere with the effect of the chemical mediators that are secondary to the immune reaction. They stop the swelling of the normal tissues, the mucous production, the inflammation, and the itching that is a result of the immune response. The pollen grains may still be there, the antibodies still produced, but the injury afforded to the surrounding tissues is reduced. The tears stop, the secretions decrease and the person can breathe again until the pollen grains are finally washed away, coughed up or no longer breathed in.

ANEMIAS, TOO, can be auto-immune. We are all familiar with one of the most common types of anemia—iron deficiency. This type is caused by a decrease in red-cell production due to insufficient iron in the diet, or to blood loss. The advertisements tell us, and it is partly true, that a few women who during their periods may bleed excessively can lose enough blood and with it enough iron to become anemic. Iron is an absolute necessity for our bone marrow to produce the hemoglobin in our circulating red cells so that these cells can do what they are supposed to do—carry oxygen to all the parts of our body. If the metal is not available, our bone marrow, like any factory whose raw materials have been cut off, simply stops its manufacture of hemoglobin, and eventually decreases its production of red cells.

But there are other kinds of anemias that have nothing to do with a lack of iron, anemias that occur when a person's red blood cells disappear mysteriously despite the fact that his body has enough iron and is even producing red cells at a gigantic rate. It can happen in patients with lupus, but it can also occur in other kinds of auto-immune disease. In these diseases transfusions don't work because no matter how often they are given, they cannot keep up with the red-cell destruction that is going on, and medications, too, prove useless. Frail, ill, easily exhausted, these patients wandered undiagnosed and untreatable until Coombs showed that they had antibodies in their serum which attacked their own red blood cells. The destruction was accomplished in the same way as the destruction of an infant's Rh-positive cells by his Rh-negative mother, except that in these patients there were no preformed antibodies delivered to their circulation. They had sensitized themselves, made antibodies against their own red cells. For some reason their red cells suddenly, after ten, twelve or twenty years, changed or were changed and their immune system read these newly changed cells as foreign.

The change may be caused by a subtle chemical alteration in the production of these cells, a mistaken addition in their manufacture by the bone marrow of an amino acid into their surface or a change in their protein configuration—caused by a poison, some dye in the food we eat, some preservative or pesticide that remains on the vegetables we consume—so that these cells are no longer antigenically normal and are therefore read as foreign as they begin to circulate. Perhaps, again, a virus somehow attaches itself to the red-cell membrane, and the two together are mistakenly read by the immune system as foreign. Whatever the origin of the trouble, these patients with the auto-immune anemias continue to suffer, and even though we know the cause of their disease, they still die because we cannot turn off their antibody production.

•　　•　　•

MULTIPLE SCLEROSIS may also be an auto-immune disease caused by antibodies the patients make against their own brain tissue. Multiple sclerosis is a disease of young adults in which a particular constituent of the brain is gradually but relentlessly destroyed. Initially the destruction was thought to be the result of a direct attack by an infecting brain virus. But the lifelong nature of multiple sclerosis, its long periods of health interspersed with episodes of paralysis, was not what would be expected from an acute infectious illness, viral, bacterial or fungal. In addition, autopsy examinations of these patients' brain showed a kind of tissue destruction different from that caused by a viral disease.

Only recently, again because of improved basic techniques in antibody research, have strange antibodies been found in the serum of multiple-sclerosis patients, auto-antibodies that seem to be made against parts of these patients' own brain, antibodies that may indeed have something to do with the production of their disease. But again, why are these antibodies produced? What, after twenty years of life, has caused these people's own brain tissue suddenly to be read as foreign and attacked by their own immune system? And why does the attack seem to stop not for days or weeks but for years, only to flare up again?

Rheumatoid arthritis, too, with its crippling deformities, is now considered to be an auto-immune disease, though different, not quite as well understood as the arthritis of children with lupus or rheumatic fever. The great majority of those suffering from rheumatoid arthritis again have a strange antibody in their bloodstream; for some inexplicable reason, these people appear literally to make antibodies against their own antibodies. Could it be that in defending themselves against infections, their own antibodies are somehow damaged in their attacks, in a sense wounded with a part lost here, something removed there, and that those damaged antibodies still circulating are read by the rest of the body's defense system as foreign and themselves attacked in turn?

These are not merely theoretical questions, to be discussed only in laboratories or behind the closed doors of international symposia. They are questions that affect all of us, for in their answers—the understanding of just how our antibodies, so much a part of us, can suddenly go astray—lies the key to much of human disease as well as the answer to our last great plague, cancer—our modern equivalent of Poe's Red Death.

15

Rejection: The Battle of Transplants

THE ANTIBODIES that patrol our vessels, the T and B lymphocytes that creep along our tissue planes, the granulocytes that will blindly attack any foreign particle, the components of complement like molecular detonators ready to blow a hole in any living thing anywhere, properdin able to cling no matter what to the surface of bacteria, histamine, serotonin, kallikrein, kinin, the body's chemical mediators capable of isolating any attacker, of walling off infections—all these are older than we are. Older by a thousand million years. They each alone proved themselves powerful, enduring and incredibly dangerous long before they moved down our own bloodstream, long before they exchanged the ancient seas for our own circulation. In the millions of years since they were trapped within us, they have protected life, made it possible for it to continue, to develop. Ultimately, they gave us the time necessary to learn to hold things and to be able to think.

The heart that beats within each of us, the idea that may linger for a summer's night or a lifetime, the desires that propel us forward or speed us backward move at the sufferance of our immune system. It sustains us all with its dedication, its single-mindedness of purpose, and suicidal heroism in the taking on of all that comes, big or small, dangerous or benign, single sentries or battalions. It never relents or backs off; it never gives up until there is nothing left to save. It will, if it has to, send in its last remaining white cell, and will, even after a billion of them have been destroyed, marshal up its last molecule of complement or properdin. It is this fanaticism that has sustained us. There is no retreat for our immune system, no moving back; only success or death, victory or defeat.

Yet like any fanatic, like any true believer, it can become destructive to the very things it aims to protect. It can destroy or maim the very thing it is sworn to defend—life itself. However much we may try to personalize our immune system, to think or feel that it shares our concerns, the truth of the matter is that it has nothing to do with our plans or wishes. It works entirely at the level of physics and chemistry, at a level so different from our human concerns, from our thinking and our feeling, our fears and desires, from even our hopes, that at times we and our immune system never meet. Nowhere is the separation more vividly illustrated than in the case of organ transplants, where the blindness of our immune system, with its autonomy, its relentless, uncompromising functioning, is not only at odds with all we wish and hope for, but where in winning its own battle, it forces us to lose ours.

There have already been over 3,000 kidney transplants performed throughout the world, 55 liver transplants, approximately 150 heart transplants, 22 lung and 30 bone-marrow transplants. Considering that in the United States alone, 9 million people suffer from kidney disease, and 100,000 annually suffer from heart disease, transplantation, or the removal of the diseased organ and its replacement by a healthy one would seem to be the answer to two of the major medical problems affecting us today. The surgeons can do it; there is no great technical skill involved in removing an organ from a healthy donor and putting it into a recipient's body. It is sheer mechanic's work. There may be some problems in organ preservation and the technical aspects of suturing together the blood supply of the recipient to the vessels of the transplant, but if that were all there was to it, transplantation would be the treatment of choice not only for heart disease and kidney failure but for liver disease and diabetes and the immunodeficiency states.

But all the original heart-transplant patients are dead now, and none of the liver or lung recipients are alive either. Kidney transplantations have become successful not because they are done differently from other transplants but because dialysis is available as a backup when they don't work right or fail. The real problem of transplantation is not technical but immunologic. What the surgeon faces is a problem not of technique or even of the will but of the body's unchanging insistence on destroying the transplanted organ, on going after it until it is rejected even if it means the body's own death. This rejection reaction is the central obstacle to all transplantation. It is an obstacle etched deep into the bitter histories of transplant patients, histories described since transplantations were first attempted, and still being published today in the world's leading medical journals.

Recently such a case—of a twenty-four-year-old man suffering from kidney disease, who had received a cadaver kidney transplant—was described in the *New England Journal of Medicine.* Coldly, dispassionately it points out the whole problem of rejection.

> The transplanted kidney produced 480 ml. of urine in the first two hours after transplantation; then the urine flow abruptly stopped. Abnormal bleeding was noticed from venapuncture sites, then profuse oozing of blood from the wound and operative surgical drains. The patient became shocky and five hours postoperative was taken back to the operating room and re-explored. When the patient's abdomen was re-opened the transplanted kidney itself was mottled in color; but still seemed grossly normal. Fresh plasma was given and the abdomen was again closed. The patient continued to do poorly and 18 hours after the original transplantation, his abdomen was again opened and re-explored. There was still excellent blood flow to the transplanted kidney, and yet despite the blood flow and the fact that the kidney itself was still in place, the surgeons found that the kidney had turned a bluish black, that it was uniformly cyanotic, soft to the touch and easily punctured. Nineteen hours

later the kidney [was dead], and had to be removed—the patient placed on dialysis.

We know by now what causes the destruction of transplanted kidneys. We know what killed the heart-transplant patients, why liver transplants never worked. When the first patients were transplanted and began rejecting their transplants, the rejected organs that had to be removed were taken back to the lab, sectioned and microscopically examined. They were found to be filled with white cells. The tissues of the rejected organ—heart, lung, liver or kidney—were completely filled with the transplant patient's own granulocytes. It was obvious to those early investigators that the recipient's white cells had flooded into the transplanted organ and attacked it, gradually destroying the organ so that it had to be removed.

Later, with ever more rejections, with more tissues to look at, with better antibody techniques, it became clear that not only were the recipient's granulocytes involved, but all of his body's other defense mechanisms. What was going on in the transplanted organ was a full-blown immune response with granulocytes, macrophages, complement, antibodies, T and B lymphocytes and properdin all taking part. Without knowing why or even how to stop the rejection, the initial transplant surgeons took comfort in at least being able to give their failures a name. They called it the "rejection phenomenon," using the words as a shield against the charges of poor judgment, of going too far too fast. It was not they, they implied, who destroyed the hearts of their heart transplants or the livers of their liver transplants, who forced their kidney patients to be wheeled down the corridor for their second or even their third transplant; it was the "rejection phenomenon." "Not our fault; we tried. It was the rejection phenomenon." "Sorry, Mrs. Brown, but the rejection phenomenon." "We'll have it licked once we get the rejection phenomenon under control."

More unrealistic hope has been generated only to be dismissed and poor judgment excused under the term "rejection phenomenon" than under any other modern scientific term except perhaps "nuclear reaction." No one doubts now that the rejection occurs. It has been scribbled on hundreds of death certificates; it is there in the faces of the dying heart recipients, written into the hopeless, knowledgeable looks of families when told again that there is no choice, that the new kidney their son or daughter has just received has failed and will have to be removed, for a time their child put back again on the dialysis machine until another kidney becomes available. Today we still use the general term "rejection phenomenon," although we know exactly what happens when a transplanted organ is placed in the recipient's body.

We knew even at the beginning of transplantations, from Landsteiner's work with blood groups and from the studies on Rh incompatibility, that red blood cells have markers—antigens —on their surface which differentiate one blood group from another. What we now know is that every cell in our body, like our red cells, have antigens on their surface, protein molecules that distinguish our own cells from the cells of anyone else. The problem is that we have "tissue group" differences between each of us as well as blood-group differences. The liver cell of your brother, even though it does the same thing for him that your liver cell does for you, has markers on its walls which are different from yours, and the same holds true for the cells that make up the tissues of your kidney and your heart, pancreas, muscles and lungs.

It is the old problem of membranes again. There would be no rejection phenomenon if the cells in the transplanted organs had the same types and arrangements of proteins in their membranes as the cells of the recipient. But they don't, and like the different antigens on the membranes of mismatched red cells which cause transfusion reactions in the recipient, the different membranes on the cells of transplanted organs cause rejections to occur. We can well ask, Why? Why the differences in cellular surfaces? Membranes don't add or detract from what cells do; they only protect what's inside. But this may be the reason for the whole problem.

We are sure that differences in membranes are under genetic control, that different types and arrangements of the proteins which go into cell-wall construction are inherited like differences in the color of our eyes, or our being tall or short. But again, why? Having blue eyes or brown has nothing to do with being able to see, or being tall or short with what kind of person one is. These variations are allowed because they have no real bearing on survival. The same applies to cellular membranes, since their structure has nothing to do with the cells' work. The evolutionary fact is that as long as one developing membrane was structurally as sound as the next, and had the correct membrane pumps, it didn't matter exactly how they were made or what proteins went into their construction. Until, that is, transfusions began and transplantation became possible. Then those differences became the difference between life and death.

When an organ is transplanted into a recipient whose genetic make-up has led to the production of tissues composed of cells with membrane antigens that differ from those antigens on the cells of the transplanted organ, it means the same to the patient's immune system as if he were suddenly attacked by a foreign organism.

Immunologically one of two things can happen when a transplanted organ with antigenically dissimilar cells is put into another person's body. In fact, both probably do. As soon as the organ is in place, tiny bits and pieces of its cells begin to break down and enter the recipient's bloodstream. This constant tissue breakdown goes on all the time, even with healthy tissues. If the antigens on the pieces of the transplanted organ were the same as the recipient's own antigens, they would be ignored, taken up by the body's waste-disposal system and removed. But with a transplanted organ they are not. Since the cells of the transplant have different surface markings than the patient's own cells, these fragments are read by the recipient's immune system as foreign; antibodies are made against them and the recipient's granulocytes begin the search for the sources of these antigens.

The other event, and probably the more common, is that the recipient's small lymphocytes, always on the alert, always moving through his circulation, eventually come in contact with the antigenically different cells of the transplant. Once in contact, they hurry back to the nearest lymph node, where they transfer the information to the B cells and the killer T lymphocytes that will eventually go out to destroy the donor organ. Indeed, on the new immunofluorescently stained microscopic sections of rejected organs, the recipient's killer lymphocytes can be seen lying right up against the foreign cells of the transplant, staying there until all those foreign cells are killed. For the kidney-transplant patient having his kidney rejected there is a substitute—dialysis. For the heart- or liver-transplant recipient there is none; those killer lymphocytes mean the patient's eventual death.

There are always two areas of attack when an immune system begins to reject a transplanted organ. The first is the antibodies' attack on the cells making up the vessels of the transplanted organ, an attack whose fixing of complement injures the cells lining these vessels. The transplanted organ's arteries and veins are clogged with the damaged and dying cells, causing the blood flow to the transplant to stop. With no blood coming to it, the organ quickly begins to die. Tissue antigens, if not released before, are released now from the millions of dying cells, more antibodies are made and the body mounts an ever more vigorous immunologic attack. The cycle is repeated and repeated, relentlessly, until the transplant, no longer supplied with blood, is nothing but dead and dying tissue.

The second area of attack is against the cells of the organ itself, not just the cells lining its blood vessels. In the case of kidney transplants, antibodies are made against the membranes on the transplanted kidney cells themselves; its tubule cells, the cells of its interstium, the glomerular cells—every kind of cell that makes up the kidney itself is attacked.

The recipient's complement is activated, his lymphocytes are turned on, macrophages and plasma cells flood into the organ. The whole kidney gradually stops functioning and is eventually destroyed.

Knowing that rejections will always occur in transplanted organs other than those whose cell surfaces exactly match the surfaces of the recipient's cells, the question has become not how to recognize these reactions but how to overcome the billion years of powerful, overwhelming chemistry that goes into that immune response. After all, what the body is doing in attacking transplanted organs is what it has been doing since life first began—protecting itself. In reality, in fighting rejection, our physicians are fighting us.

"What is his serum creatinine?" Dr. Kelder asks.

"It was one point two."

"I didn't ask what it was," Kelder says, annoyed, "I asked what it is."

"Two point one today," the intern answers.

"Then his kidney function is definitely getting worse."

Kelder looks at the blood-chemistry flow sheet tacked up on the wall. The chief transplant resident, still in his surgical greens, stands relaxed behind the mobile chart rack; he is the only one in the group who is not tense. The intern, the first- and second-year residents, the dialysis group, and the students around the chart rack all stand more or less at attention, looking nervously at Kelder, waiting for him to say something, to ask a question, demand an answer. Even the nurses passing become quiet; they stop talking and walk more softly, until they are safely by.

"How long postransplant is he?" Kelder asks.

"Five months," the intern says.

"Didn't he have some trouble immediate posttransplant?"

The intern looks nervously at Clark, the chief resident. "Yes," Clark answers for the intern. "He had some acute tubular necrosis. He had to be dialyzed for two or three weeks, then his kidney opened up and he finally started putting out urine."

"Did he get ALG?"

"Yes," Clark replies. "We were using it then. It was part of the transplant protocol, it was being given to any recipient getting less than an A matched transplant."

Kelder frowns and looks back at the group. "And the donor?"

"A cadaver kidney," Clark says. "There were no related donors available. The mother and her brother would have been donors but they were incompatible, different major blood types. The parents were divorced and the father who was compatible refused to be a donor. Something about his new wife refusing to let him give a kidney to his son, or not being able to take time off work . . . something like that."

Kelder gives no sign he has heard the last remark. He looks at the chart once more, then walks quickly into the patient's room. The students hesitate. Stepping away from the chart rack, Clark motions them to follow and walks with them into the room. Kelder is already talking to the patient, who is sitting propped up in bed.

"You're doing fine," Kelder says.

For those not accustomed to seeing transplant patients, the comment would seem blind, if not foolish. The patient looks ill, his face is round, almost grotesquely moonlike, from his anti-rejection medication. His arms, sticking out from under the covers, are thin-looking, wasted. There are bruises all over his body, black and blue spots up and down his chest and along his neck. He is having trouble breathing, taking short little gasps.

"We think your kidney will be okay," Kelder says. The patient looks relieved. Kelder pats him on the knees and leaves with the group following him.

"How much steroid is he on?" he asks when they are outside the room.

"Sixty milligrams prednisone," the intern answers.

"And Imuran?"

"Three milligrams per kilo, once a day."

"Well, jack it up and give him Solucortef. Give him the whole rejection therapy."

Clark looks disturbed. "But he still has that infiltrate in his lung, and a fever. It might not be a rejection. The biopsy we did yesterday on his kidney wasn't much help. There was nothing specific there," he cautions, "just a few lymphocytes near some of the tubule cells."

"Did any of the cultures grow out anything?" Kelder asks.

"No, they didn't, not yet anyway. But I still think that—"

Kelder's face sets. "Any titers back against CID or any of the other viral infections?" he asks coldly.

"Not yet."

"Blood cultures, urine cultures, throat cultures grow out anything? Sputum cultures?"

"No, not yet, they're all still negative, but—"

"Then the fever could be from his rejection. Right?"

"Yes, but—"

"Then you better treat him for rejection."

"But even without the fever, his kidney function could be getting worse because of an infection."

"Treat him for rejection . . . and right now."

That afternoon they begin giving the patient more steroids,

massive doses, and more Imuran, and take him to X-ray to radiate his kidney. It is not often that a chief resident in surgery questions, much less challenges, the head of his department, but Clark and Kelder were not arguing about medications or procedures; they were talking about life and death. The two physicians, resident and chief, could be at odds here because when it came to the question of whether to treat the patient's fever and decreasing kidney function as a rejection episode or as an infection, they were speaking as equals; neither really knew if he was right. And both knew that if they were wrong, they would be killing the patient.

THE BODY'S IMMUNE defenses can be muted. Today we have drugs that in essence poison the body's immune system and can destroy a billion years of defenses in a few days, or if necessary, in a few hours. These chemical immunosuppressives have in no small measure been responsible for what success there has been in the field of transplantation. Most of these drugs were derived from cancer chemotherapy. They had proved their worth in interfering with abnormal cancerous cellular division, and were then adopted by the transplantation specialists to suppress the immune responses.

For years, immunologists had realized that the incredible effectiveness of our immune system resides in part in its ability to respond so massively to any attacker. The cells that make up the system—the plasma cells in our bone marrow and the lymph nodes constantly making the millions of necessary antibodies, the billions of white cells available to be thrown at any moment into the battle, with millions more to come later, the small lymphocytes constantly patrolling our vessels, ready to process any antigen, the rapid proliferation of thousands of killer lymphocytes from seemingly silent lymph nodes—all make the immune system the most metabolically active system in our bodies.

Because of the similarities in the rapid proliferations and increased metabolic activities of the immune cells which provide the tools for our protection, with the increased metabolic rate and rapid growth of cancer cells, our immune system will, like cancer, take up drugs faster than the other, less active tissues of the body. Because of this increased pickup rate, both our immune system and cancer cells will become poisoned on doses of a drug well below the levels needed to poison the other cells of the body, so much lower that these dangerous drugs can be given in small amounts that will affect only them while sparing other, less active tissues. This difference in drug uptake becomes the rationale not only for cancer therapy but also the basis of treatment for rejection.

The immunosuppressive drugs get into the cells dividing to form our granulocytes, and into the plasma cells forming our antibodies, and poison them. They keep immature lymphocytes from differentiating into T and B cells, and antigens brought back to lymph nodes from being processed. The drugs work; the immune response can be poisoned, its attacks on transplanted organs can be stopped. But there is no such thing as destroying only the white cells and antibodies directed against an antigen on a foreign kidney cell's surface or those that go after a heart transplant; the whole immune system is affected. We can't just poison one part of the immune response. If we mute its attack against a transplanted organ, we also of necessity poison its ability to attack any real foreign invader, any attacking bacteria or viruses.

That is the price we pay, and it was what worried Clark and what he and Kelder were really arguing about. Even the ALG that Clark said had been given is a nonspecific immunosuppressive. ALG are the letters that stand for Antilymphocyte globulin. It is made by injecting a horse with human lymphocytes. The horse makes antibodies against these human lymphocytes. Blood is then removed from the horse, the globulin fraction which contains all the horse's antibodies is separated, and the portion containing the antibodies to human lymphocytes is given intravenously to the patient about to receive a transplant. The aim is to destroy the lymphocytes in the recipient's circulation so that none will be left to process the foreign antigens on the cells of the transplanted organ once it is placed in the body.

But again, it is not one group of lymphocytes—those that will eventually attack the transplant—which are destroyed, but all the recipient's lymphocytes. It is possible with ALG to drop a person's lymphocyte count from 6,000 per cubic milliliter of his blood to zero, to deplete his circulating lymphocytes so that none are left. By using all of it—ALG, steroids and Imuran—the rejection phenomenon can be stopped but so will the rest of the body's defenses, leaving those immunosuppressed as helpless as the infant born without any immune system at all.

When Clark cautioned about the chest X-ray showing something in the patient's lungs, what he was warning was that if that something was a pneumonia, and if they gave the patient more immunosuppressive therapy, the pneumonia would spread. With the body's immune system poisoned, the bacteria or viruses in the patient's chest, no longer kept under control by his own white cells and antibodies, would spread quickly throughout his lungs and then eventually out into his whole body. If it was not a rejection causing the decrease in the patient's kidney function, as well as his fever, but an infection, and the immunosuppressive drugs were increased, the patient would go on to die from his infection. The fact that the patient was already on maintenance immunosuppressive drugs made the problem of infection even a greater consideration. Still, if they were wrong, and the patient was undergoing a rejection, withholding treatment would cause him to lose his kidney.

Neither Clark nor Kelder could be sure; the question had no answer. Increase the immunosuppression and stop the rejection but leave the patient open to dying from a possible infection, or decrease the drugs and give the patient a chance to fight his infection, but lose his kidney. It happens all the time, and as many times as the surgeons guess right, they guess wrong.

Today we know that as powerful as our immune system is in protecting us, it can be equally powerful and relentless in pursuing our destruction. We have only recently begun to realize that each click of the immune clock ticking within us means another second of life, gives each of us another moment to live and breathe, to run and enjoy, to love or to hate. But we have also come to realize that the clock can begin ticking out our end, not only for organs that have been transplanted but for those we normally carry within us, those that we had thought, and indeed were, healthy before our immune system turned on them.

16

Cancer

CANCER IS a disease of aging. Many cancers are ultimately caused by environmental poisons, like food preservatives and cigarette smoking, a few are probably caused by viruses, but most, whatever the cause, do not appear until we get older. Cancer has always been a dreaded part of human disease, and people have always died from it, but not in the astonishing numbers of today. The statisticians tell us that the increase in cancer cases has nothing to do with changes in the disease itself; that the cancers we see today are the ones we've always seen; that only the numbers, attack rates and susceptibilities are different.

Its increase seems in part to be a result of medicine's successes with the infectious diseases, with its development of vaccines and antibiotics. People who used to die of pneumonias and meningitis, of measles and polio, of peritonitis and wound infections, survive today; children with rheumatic fever, who used to be dead before their teens of rheumatic heart disease, no longer die; people with third-degree burns, which used to be fatal, survive; most young mothers now come home healthy after their deliveries; occluded coronary arteries can be fixed, cardiac arrhythmias and hypertension controlled. Accident victims given IV's at the roadside are no longer brought into emergency rooms dead; wounded soldiers are medevacked within minutes of being hit. We live longer today, and it is because of this that the incidence of cancer goes up. Survival and the aging that goes with it seem to be the cause.

Why? What goes wrong and why does it lead to cancer? Why will one out of fourteen women after forty or fifty years of life have to have a breast removed? Why will 50 percent of all men, if they live long enough, have their prostates turn cancerous? Why? We think today we know the answer, and while it is not very pleasant, it is not hopeless, either, at least not totally. There are young researchers working now to cure cancer, as Jenner and Pasteur once worked to cure smallpox and rabies, and while their successes may well be too late for many of us, as those of Jenner and Pasteur were already too late for many of their own contemporaries, they may not be so for our children. There should be great comfort in that.

The answer to cancers lies in stopping exposures to cancer-causing poisons, but the whys relating cancer to aging goes back again to our immune system, and what we have come to call immune surveillance.

Our bodies are made up of over a trillion individual cells, all of which have learned through the long process of evolution to work together, to maintain one another, to do what they do and yet support the whole, so that each will in turn be maintained and protected. Our body is like a great movable city, made up of a trillion individuals all with different skills, yet working together. It has its own ventilation and sewage systems, its own telephone and communications network, a billion miles of interconnecting highways and side streets, a system of alleys, its own supermarkets and factories, disposal plants and heating units. All it really needs to keep going are a few basic raw materials to be brought in—sugars, fats, proteins, carbon, hydrogen, oxygen, nitrogen, magnesium, iron, zinc and calcium, and a way of discharging wastes.

Yet, as with any city, there can be natural disasters. Sewers can be clogged, arteries and water mains can rupture, the communications system can become jumbled or short-circuited, ventilation can break down, or even more important, there can be anarchy and crime. In some narrow side street or back alley, at the end of the spleen or in the outer part of the lung, a person or a cell can suddenly go bad, and forgetting or brushing off the civilized restraints, come to think only of itself, its own needs.

Like any beginning conspiracy, at first there is very little noticeable change. Things go on as they always have; the person or the cell continue outwardly to perform as they always have. Yet something is happening. The man still working in the factory continues to twist the bolts, the cell in the liver still produces the right enzyme or protein. But the bolt isn't tightened quite right and the protein's structure is slightly off, the enzyme a little less effective. Since the flawed products are mixed in with all the normal products, no one notices. But the conspiracy grows; more cells change. The neighbors may even become frightened, but remain silent.

If there were no police, there would eventually be no city. Criminals, conspiracies and individual self-service would be the rule. There would be no order in which commerce could go on, no structure for justice; it would all be chaos. The abnormal cells would, like criminals, eventually siphon off all the body's energy and all its resources. After a time, robbed and cheated, the body like the city would, simply fall apart and die.

We both need a police force; our body's is our immune system. Like the police who cruise the neighborhoods of Baltimore and Chicago, New York and Cleveland, trying to pick up individual criminals and contain gangs before they get out of control, to stop conspiracies before they have the time to gather such force that the only real answer then becomes devastating, relentless war in which the city as well as the criminals would be destroyed, our immune police, our lymphocytes and antibodies, patrol the body trying to find abnormal cells and cancerous conspiracies before they grow large enough to cause real harm. Both try to stop anarchy before it becomes riot, disease before it becomes rebellion.

It has been known for over a hundred years, ever since the discovery of antibodies in the late nineteenth century, that our immune system is absolutely necessary to protect us from bacteria and viruses. But it was not until the late nineteen-sixties that Burnett, an Australian, offered a theory so new and so different that it is still being debated today. He proposed that our immune system protects us not only from outside invaders but from those inside as well.

Our body is not static; we produce a whole new layer of skin once every ten days, our bone marrow continually pumps new red cells and white cells into our circulation, the linings of our stomach and intestines are continually being replaced. Every hour the cells covering our eyes are washed away in our tears, only to have others exactly like them take their place. Our hair and nails keep breaking off, but more are always formed. Our testes produce billions of new sperm each day, and our ovaries are supplied with an almost unlimited number of eggs. Our body is always replacing itself; for every cell that is lost or used up, a new one exactly like it takes its place. The replicating process that brings it all about is as old as life itself, and goes back to how life first renewed itself; indeed, it *is* life.

No matter how it is done, in whatever way this replication takes place, it is still a purely physical process. Membranes have to be exactly copied, new ones precisely like the old have to be produced; nuclei have to be copied one from the other; the precise sequence of cellular enzymes and proteins must be rigorously maintained; and all this not just once but millions of times a day, and not just one day but every day of our lives.

Simple mechanical mistakes occur: an enzyme is bound to be occasionally missed, a membrane not copied exactly right, the nuclei a little off center, a protein one amino acid off. In those ancient seas, the mistakes simply died, or if the new product was slightly better suited to the environment, it survived and was passed on. One way or the other, the mistakes of replication were of no concern to nature; the new cells either died or started a whole new line of better-suited, more effective cells that carried evolution forward another step.

But in the internal economy of the body, where each cell depends on the one next to it, where demands for mutual interaction and dependency have become so strict that no mistakes can be tolerated, these abnormal cells must be destroyed. We need our liver to do what livers do—store and release sugars for other parts of the body to use as fuel, to detoxify our internal poisons, to purify the products coming from other organs, to make the proteins that other cells need for bodily repairs. We need our brain cells to think and move our body; our heart cells to pump our blood. Our body cannot tolerate any of its cells going off on their own, ignoring their normal functions as they grow and divide, concerned only with their own survival, their own individual replication.

Burnett realized that the body, in reproducing its billions of new cells daily, must in the course of those twenty-four hours commit not just one error of replication, but many; and that during one day alone, from ten to a hundred abnormal, independent, potentially cancerous cells might be produced. He felt sure that our immune system—with its antibodies everywhere in the bloodstream and tissue fluids, its white cells and lymphocytes in the course of their unending patrols, literally touching every living cell, its macrophages that sit in virtually every organ, even the brain—was the only system we had capable of recognizing these abnormal cells as foreign and going after them with the same homicidal grimness that it goes after any bacteria, viruses or protozoa, destroying these mistakes as it does the microbes, killing them, as it does bacteria and viruses, before they can divide and grow. How else, Burnett reasoned, are we not all taken over by these cells?

In his theory, Burnett went on to state that for the most part our immune system is successful; each abnormal cell—whenever and wherever it arises, in muscle, liver, brain or lung—is discovered by our immune system, attacked and destroyed. It is how we have managed to survive; indeed, this internal control is as crucial to our survival as is our ability to fight outside attackers. But, he warned, if anything happens to our immune system, if there is any weakening of its ability to recognize these abnormal cells or to destroy them, they will grow and become cancers. No longer under the normal restraints of division and growth, these cells will gradually take over the organ in which they arose, replacing the normal cells with their own, stopping the organ from performing its necessary function. If this happens in an organ that is absolutely necessary—like the lungs for breathing or the kidneys for eliminating our wastes, the liver for detoxification and fuel—the person will die when enough of that organ is taken over. If the organ is not that crucial, the cancer will continue to grow, sometimes spreading to other organs, killing the patient slowly, by degrees.

Burnett's theory about how cancer begins may be questioned, his theory can be argued, but not what happens after the cancer is once established. What happens then has already been unarguably entered in thousands of medical records and in the hearts and minds of millions of friends and relatives.

OCTOBER 19: *Medical progress note. Diagnosis: Lung cancer. Biopsy diagnosis: Bronchial biopsy, squamous cell carcinoma; metastatic spread to bone and liver.*

"It was just a routine physical, the doctor took a chest X-ray and saw this shadow near the top of his lung. He sent us to a thoracic surgeon who tried to be nice, but we knew. He said that Herb needed a biopsy and so we had him admitted to the hospital the next day, and they did a biopsy. It was lung cancer."

OCTOBER 20: *Due to severe unrelenting bone pain, have increased Demerol . . . new bony lesions of the spine, lumbar vertebrae L1 and L2, visual on X-ray bone survey.*

"Herb took it very well. Dr. Brown said that if things went well, Herb would have six to eight months. . . . We talked and Herb said how lucky he really was to have time to put all his things in order . . . that . . . that many men don't have that. He talked of a few people he knew, businessmen, who had had heart attacks without . . . without . . ."

NOVEMBER 9: *Erosion of lumbar spines have continued with neurological involvement of spinal cord. Patient now has loss of rectal and bladder function; neurosurgeons consulted. Their recommendation due to patient's terminal condition is to do nothing. Patient becoming hostile; have changed pain medication from Demerol to morphine.*

"It's difficult to know now what was really the hardest. I think if it would have lasted much longer, we would have really had trouble with our oldest boy; towards the end, he stopped studying and would just sit in his room. Our youngest child was first bewildered and I think angry that I was spending so much time at the hospital."

NOVEMBER 16: *The patient is unable to keep down any food. Have begun IV therapy, patient is becoming very withdrawn.*

"And to tell you the horrible truth, at the end I could barely bring myself to even walk into his room; don't think poorly of me, please don't, but once, just once, I didn't go. . . . I stayed home . . . he looked so terrible and tried so hard to show how it didn't hurt . . . I just stayed home and cried . . ."

———————

HOW DOES IT BEGIN? Why do cancers grow? Those are the questions. For cures we have to know causes. The answer for polio, as we all know, was not a better iron lung, but learning what caused the paralysis, discovering the virus that did it, growing the virus and then making the vaccine. We must know the causes, the beginning of a disease, before we can act, and now with more and more cancer research being done and more and more observations of cancers themselves, researchers have begun to think that Burnett is right. Some have become so sure about the importance of our immune system in allowing the beginning of cancer that like Good, who became a leader in the field of immunology by refusing to back down about the cause of auto-immune diseases, they too are now willing to state definitely that "in order for cancer to occur and persist, there must be a failure of the immune processes, either in surveillance or destruction."

In short, we are the ones who allow our own cancers to develop; that cells once undergoing malignant transformations grow because of a failure of our immune system to protect us. A great deal of evidence points to this. The first and most obvious fact is that cancers occur most commonly in the very young and the very old, two groups in which the immune system either has not yet reached full development or has begun to wear out. We know that newborns cannot mount as effective an immune response as adults can, and that with age our immune response simply loses its potency.

There has never been much research done on aging. It may

have been too hard to do, or simply not been fashionable; more likely, though, was the fact that it lacked the excitement of acute medical research—the prestige that went into the development of open-heart surgery, the drama of lowering of blood pressures with drugs. The control of cardiac arrhythmia with nickel cadmium-powered pacemakers and the discoveries of ever newer and more powerful antibiotics are what held people's interest. But recently, under the pressures of trying to prove or disprove Burnett's theory of immune surveillance, work has finally begun on the aging process itself.

This work has yielded some startling and depressing discoveries, with unpleasant implications for all of us. Recent studies have shown that the antibody response of old mice declines to about 5 percent of the values of the same mice tested when younger. Cellular immune responses universally decline with age to a fourth or less of their value in younger animals, no matter what the species, and humans as well. These are apparently unalterable immunologic facts, and their implications in regard to our body's protecting itself from a continually developing supply of potentially cancerous cells are obvious, if not conclusive.

Most evidence concerning the depression of our immune system and the development of cancer has come from humans who have had to be put on drugs that suppress their immune responses. Rejection therapy in kidney-transplant patients is an absolute necessity if we want their transplanted organs to survive. Immunosuppressive drugs which interfere with the transplant recipient's antibody synthesis, his white-cell functions, must be given until the new organ is finally, if ever, accepted. Yet the suppression of the transplant's immunologic system is not a specific suppression, restricted just to his newly transplanted organ. It is a general suppression that will affect the patient's immune response to any foreign substance. While on high doses of these immunosuppressive drugs, the transplant patient's body is more susceptible to bacterial and viral infections than it would normally be. Accordingly, the transplant surgeons reduce the dosage of these drugs as soon as they can, but many patients, because of a continuing low-grade chronic rejection, have to be maintained on tiny but continuous dosages

—dosages that stop their rejections but are not high enough to interfere with their body's fighting off attacks of bacteria or viruses.

If Burnett was right, if immune surveillance is important in retarding or preventing cancerous growths, then you would expect to find more cancers in younger people who have had their immune systems interfered with artificially than nonsuppressed people their own age, just as we find more cancers in older people who have had their immune surveillance interfered with naturally.

These young transplant patients, with their immune systems suppressed, were in a sense an already developed experimental group exactly suited to test Burnett's theory, and when they were studied, the results did indeed tend to support his theory. The National Institutes of Health studied 8,000 transplant patients and found 777 cases of cancer. The incidence of cancer in these immunologically suppressed patients was over a hundred times the incidence of naturally occurring cancer in people of their same age group in the general population. Even more important was the fact that the cancers which occurred in these suffering transplant patients were, for the most part, cell for cell, like cancers seen only in older people.

Children, too—those with lupus and the other autoimmune hemolytic anemias who had to be put on immunosuppressive medications to decrease their production of antibodies in order to stop or slow their own disease—were also found to have developed a small but significantly important number of bizarre and totally unexpected brain and bone-marrow malignancies which were never seen before in children of their age, and never in those places within their bodies.

A certain kind of mice called the NZB strain—all of which, like the Aleutian mink, have a defect in their immune system —develop tumors, cancers of the skin and gut. On the other hand, normal mice without this defect—apparently with their immune ability still intact and so able to destroy any abnormal, potentially cancerous cell that might be formed within them— do not. The only thing wrong with the cancerous NZB strain is a defect in their immune system, nothing else.

But on purely scientific grounds, the unequivocal evidence —that a defect in immune surveillance is the cause of cancer growth—has not yet been found. Cancer research, groping around in the dark for a definitive answer, is still giving confusing and conflicting results about immune surveillance. A recent large body of independent evidence has begun to indicate that cancer might well be caused by more than a defect in immune surveillance.

It was proposed by other researchers that the ability to mount an immune response to a foreign substance is genetically predetermined and has nothing to do with the intactness of the immune system itself. After all, they reasoned, arguing against Burnett, only 60 to 70 percent of healthy Rh-negative, immunologically perfect volunteers, when injected with Rh-positive cells, developed Rh-positive antibodies; and going further, they reasoned, only a small number of individuals ever acquire hay fever, even though everyone is exposed to the same pollen grains. Studies have shown that some people with an obviously adequate functioning immune system, with everything perfectly intact, still cannot respond to a large number of injected foreign antigens. It is not, the researchers proposed, just a defect in immune surveillance that leads to cancer growth, but something else—genetics itself.

These scientists went on to make an important observation supporting their genetic theory: in those people suffering from naturally occurring, though minimal immunologic defects, specific defects were associated with specific types of malignancies. Patients with an inability to make some kinds of antibodies were found to be those suffering and dying from chronic lymphocytic leukemia and multiple myelomas, two very specific kinds of cancer, while patients with cancer of the colon, lung cancer, and cancers of the liver and kidney, the so-called solid metastatic tumors, were people who could make antibodies, but were found to have a minor defect in their cellular immunity, in their T and B lymphocytes. If cancers are caused by a general, nonspecific defect in overall immune surveillance, they said, then why weren't these patients having all kinds of cancer rather than just specific ones?

The attack on Burnett's theory continued. The more that cancers were studied, the more it became clear that many first begin as precancerous lesions which can and do exist for years before the real cancers emerge from them. Physicians have long been aware that leukoplakic change in the epidermis precedes invasive squamous cell carcinoma of the skin; lentigo maligna precedes frank malignant melanoma; intestinal polyps precede cancer of the colon; benign hydatidiform moles grow into choriocarcinoma.

Despite the abnormal, precancerous cells being present and continually exposed to the patient's immune surveillance system for long periods of time, no immune response is mounted against them, nor is an immune response ever begun, even when the precancerous sores become overtly cancerous. It was proposed that in these tumors, some of the most malignant on earth, immune surveillance plays no part, that the cells turn cancerous and begin to take over the person's body simply when they "feel" like it or have existed long enough to precipitate intracellular disruptions to such a degree that the cells finally so greatly changed take off on their own, unapprehendable criminals free to do as they please.

Other scientists have found blocking antibodies, or combinations of tumor antigens with anti-tumor antibodies, circulating in the blood of cancer patients. It has been proposed that these antigen-antibody complexes interfere with the patient's immune system by binding up his antibodies in the circulation before they can even reach the tumor and begin their attack. These researchers suggest it is not defective immune surveillance that allows a cancer to grow, but the body's being fooled by circulating tumor antigens into wasting itself on these decoys, making the fight in the bloodstream instead of where it should, in the tissues, on the cancer cells themselves. It may be that sometimes our body is our own worst enemy, making antibodies that decoy all the rest of our immune system into making the wrong fight in the wrong place, or that the tumors are cleverer than we care to admit.

Others have proposed that as cancer grows—whether in our lungs or kidneys, breasts or ovaries—our normal blood vessels grow with them, supplying what they still think is normal tissue with the needed oxygen and food. This ingrowth of normal vessels could establish a barrier between the foreign cancer and our own immune system, in a sense protecting the tumor by fooling the immune system into thinking there is nothing foreign or dangerous there on the other side of that normal vessel wall.

Tumors have also been described that seem to have no antigens on their surface at all. Cancers produced by "carcinogens," or chemical poisons like food preservatives or cigarette smoke, seem to be of this kind. Immune surveillance here would mean nothing one way or the other. With no antigens on these cancer cells, no surface to be read as foreign, the cancers take hold and continue to grow unhindered even in people with normal immune systems because the cancerous cells have nothing on them to be read as foreign.

The arguments still rage. At the 1970 International Symposium of Immunology the proponents of the blocking-antibody theory of cancer growth were shouted down by the immune-surveillance proponents, while followers of the non-antigen theory fought with both groups.

IN 1968, as a result of a tragic mistake, the importance of the immune system in combating and controlling cancer was established beyond dispute. For the first time in over six years of successful kidney transplants, a cancerous kidney was placed in an immunologically suppressed person. Of course the surgeons involved didn't know there was cancer in the transplanted kidney; they had done everything possible, as they always do, to make sure that the donor kidney was normal. But there is no way to pick up small tumors in the center of normal-looking kidneys if the cancer has not grown large enough to show itself. There may be only one or two cells present that are cancerous, a little nodule unobserved and unobservable. If the cancer, any cancer, is smaller than half a centimeter in diameter, no medical tests—radioactive injections or arterial angiograms—will show it.

The kidney used in this transplantation was, from all studies and all observations, perfectly normal. After the transplant the patient was put on the routine high doses of anti-rejection immunosuppressive drugs. Within days the transplanted kidney began to enlarge; it looked as if there were some kind of acute rejection going on, some abnormal response, but the kidney's function remained normal. A few days later on a routine chest

X-ray, a mass was found in the patient's chest. It hadn't been there on earlier chest films, some taken as close as four days before, and it didn't have the contour of a pneumonia or some other infectious process; it was definitely a tumor. But how could it have been there and grown so large when just days before, the patient's chest had been normal?

A day later another mass was seen in the other lung field. The patient was taken back to the operating room, and when the abdomen was opened the transplanted kidney was found to have its upper half three times the size of its lower half. When this abnormal upper pole was biopsied, the frozen section showed cancer. It was then assumed that the masses in the patient's lungs were metastatic cancer that had spread from the cancer in the kidney. The physicians were startled at how fast it had spread and grown. Within days a kidney cancer that usually takes months, if not years, to become evident in the kidney itself had literally taken over this patient, metastasizing to his lungs while causing the kidney to grow to three times its normal size. The doctors had no choice but to stop all immunosuppressive therapy.

Again within days, as the patient's immune system came back to normal, the masses in his lungs began to disappear and his transplanted kidney began to shrink in size. But with the stoppage of the drugs, it became obvious to the physicians that as the patient began to "reject" his cancerous cells, he also began to reject his transplanted kidney. They had no choice. They could not run the risk of the cancer returning, so they kept the patient off his immunosuppressive drugs; the cancer was destroyed but the kidney was also completely rejected. The rejected kidney was removed and the patient put back on chronic dialysis. He survived with no further evidence of cancer.

The physicians postulated from this potentially terrifying case that the immune system of the original donor had kept the tumor that was in his own kidney from growing and getting out of hand, but that once transplanted into the recipient, who was having his immune system suppressed by the anti-rejection medications, the tumor no longer restricted by an immune system began to grow, not only to grow, but to spread throughout its new host's body. It appeared that by stopping the immunosuppressive medications and letting the recipient's immune system come back to normal, he was able to fight off the cancer, but in the process he went on to reject his transplanted kidney, too. In the real world of physics and chemistry, you cannot have it both ways.

Doctors who treat cancer patients accepted what happened with the transplanted patient as proof of the importance of the immune system in fighting malignancies. They then began to look for ways to bring the immune system of their own cancer patients into play; to gear up the system, even if still normal, to make an even better fight. Just as Jenner and Pasteur, Salk and Enders had used the body's immune system to conquer infectious diseases, this new generation of doctors began trying to use it to conquer cancer.

They have not yet been fully successful, but there is hope. Physicians and surgeons are no longer stumbling around blindly. They have a path to try, and for better or worse, they are getting on with it. If the studies and the theories that gave rise to these new procedures are correct, showing that the failure of the immune system is indeed somehow involved with either the beginnings of cancer or its continuing growth and spread, then any condition that would gear up the system should help destroy or at least retard the spread of cancerous growths.

Researchers began to re-examine what had been reported as spontaneous cures of cancer. When they reviewed the original reports they found that those patients who had had the tumor regressions all had them after having contracted and survived a severe bacterial infection.

The connection between infection and cancer cures had been reported earlier. Coley, an Englishman, in the nineteenth century, reported having stood by the bedside of a dying patient and watched as an inoperable sarcoma, a cancer of the muscle, regressed following a severe strep infection of the skin that had occurred on and near the tumor site itself. Fifty years ahead of everyone else, Coley went on to publish papers on his attempts to cure other cancer victims by injecting them with a mixture of dead and toxic bacterial cells and products. At the time he knew nothing of the mechanisms involved; his efforts to cure cancer by injecting bacterial toxins occurred long before the discovery of the four classes of antibody—the T and B lymphocytes, complement and properdin—before there was any concept at all of immune surveillance. There are suggestions here and there in his papers of occasional therapeutic responses, but the work was too ill-defined, in a sense too hopeful, without adequate controls to draw any definitive therapeutic conclusions. Still, there was a hint of possible success, and fifty years later, when his papers were reread, that hint was sufficient for those who read them.

In the sixties, researchers following Coley's lead began to use newly available materials that when injected were known to heighten an animal's immune response. One of the materials they used was called BCG (for Bacillus Calmette-Guérin), a live bacterium related to the bacillus that causes tuberculosis. Indeed, forty years ago it *was* the tubercle bacillus, but after thirteen years of growing and regrowing it in a special broth, Calmette and Guérin, two French immunologists, finally changed it into a bacillus that had lost its disease-producing properties, yet was still close enough to the original tubercle bacillus to be used throughout the world as a vaccine against tuberculosis.

Cancer researchers began using this BCG in their experiments. They removed tumors from cancerous mice and injected the tumor cells into healthy mice, also into those that had been previously inoculated with the live BCG bacillus. The results were fairly conclusive. Forty-five percent of those mice infected with the BCG before being given the cancer cells were able to inhibit the growth of the injected tumors, while those not given BCG could not. But it also appeared that in 10 percent of the BCG-infected mice, the injected cancer for some reason grew faster than in those not previously infected. Additional work on tumor growth in BCG-infected mice, rats, hamsters and guinea pigs confirmed these first observations—that pre-treatment with BCG could in about half the cases gear up the immune system of these pre-treated mice to inhibit the cancerous growths. This wasn't very good, but half of anything when the whole thing is death was enough incentive for the researchers to keep going. Plainly, pre-infection with BCG had stimulated the animals' immune response to fight the bacillus, and their heightened immune ability had also allowed them to go after the antigens on the injected cancer cells more effectively.

Scientists looked for other verification that stimulation of the immune response retarded cancers and found it in an unexpected source and in an unexpected area: Quebec, Canada. In Quebec it is government policy that all children be immunized with BCG as prevention against tuberculosis. No one is excluded. The medical records seemed to indicate that there was a decreased incidence of childhood leukemia in these immunized children when compared with children in other countries who were not required to be immunized with BCG. Following these leads, scientists at UCLA used BCG to increase the immune response in patients suffering from malignant melanomas of the skin. Some patients, but not all, have been cured by the treatment, free of disease for two years or more.

The fact that cancer is a world-wide disease has made the effort to control it a world-wide struggle. In France in the late sixties, Georges Mathe injected BCG into a child dying of leukemia. This first use of immunotherapy in leukemia resulted in a good, though partial clinical response; the patient improved, but died later from his leukemia. Mathe, encouraged by this partial success, improved his immunologic procedure. He started treating other leukemic children, first with chemotherapy, quickly reducing the number of leukemic cells in their bloodstream from billions to less than one hundred thousand. He then combined his BCG with dead tumor cells similar to leukemic cells of his patients and injected both together into these already chemo-treated children, trying to gear up their immune system to be able to hunt down those last hundred thousand cells and destroy them, wherever they might be, to get the last leukemic cell, something that chemotherapy itself had never been able to do. He was more successful, but there is some doubt now whether his success was due to BCG and its enhancement of these children's immune responses toward the antigens on their remaining leukemic cells or merely to the type of patients he had selected for treatment.

Here in America, Kelins found that by putting various irritating chemicals around the borders of some skin cancers, he could cause a severe allergic reaction at the tumor site, and with the beginnings of this reaction that some of the tumors would disappear. He reasoned that the chemical irritant had, like

BCG, caused the patient's immune system to gear up and that when it launched an attack on the applied chemical, an attack that showed itself as a severe allergic skin reaction at the application site it also went after the nearby cancer. Kelin now claims that 95 percent of his skin-cancer patients have been permanently cured. Other researchers following Kelin's ideas injected antigens directly into the tumors themselves. In some, these injections have caused tumor regression, but in others they have somehow enhanced the tumor growths, causing rapid metastatic spread and uncontrollable growths of the primaries.

There is some fear now that the growth of tumors, in areas other than around tumor sites injected with BCG or spread over with a covering of irritating chemicals, is caused by massive release of tumor antigens into the circulation and by the production of blocking antibodies. It appears that the production of these antibodies is similar to those produced in some of the earlier mice experiments which routinely caused the 10 percent infected with BCG to have accelerated tumor growth and more rapid death rather than cancer cures following tumor injections. There is some thought now that spontaneous cures of cancer have occurred not only in response to infections, as had been proposed, but also in response to spontaneous decreases in these blocking antibodies. A reduction in a cancerous person's circulating blocking antibodies, a lowering of his level of blocking antibodies, could let his immune system go after the tumor cells themselves.

The great question today remains how to bring about spontaneous cures for all people with cancer. It is a question whose answer must go back to the brutal realities of the first warm seas. Then as now, it is not sufficient to get rid of 90 percent or even 99 percent of any newly developing abnormal cells. The pressures to live, to grow, to divide, to rule, the force that has always driven life to persist and survive, are just too great. Every newly abnormal cell must be destroyed, each and every one must be hunted down and killed. If just one is left anywhere, it will grow again and again, until it finally wins. One thing is certain—once cancer begins, it is only immunology that can give us the tools necessary to make the fight that might eventually let us win.

Today in our confusion about cancer, in our lack of fundamental understanding about how it really begins, why it grows, how it can be controlled, and finally how it can be cured, we stand where we once stood in regard to infectious diseases. And we can be sure that the same things that happened with infectious-disease research will happen again here. Wrong theories will be proposed, dead ends followed, inadequate treatments championed and trumpeted. But as with the infectious plagues, in the end we shall win. And the ultimate victory, as with polio and measles, will in reality have nothing to do with an understanding of the mechanisms of cellular proliferation or the ability to unblock antibodies or even to improve our own immune systems, but with prevention.

The final answer, whatever it is, will not be concerned with destroying cancerous cells, but with the stopping of normal cells from becoming cancerous in the first place. Many cancers might be so poorly antigenic themselves, have membranes so little changed from normal cells that the body's immune system, even stimulated, could never hunt them down or even find them, nor would the removal of blocking antibodies, even if they existed, be of any benefit at all.

For these cancers, even more than the others, there can be no answer but prevention, and for that we can already begin. There is enough accumulated evidence, no matter how vague any one individual piece of it may be, to force us as prudent, caring men and women to do something now to save ourselves and keep our children from the sufferings of cancer, from the pain of having their lungs eaten away or the stomach slowly destroyed.

We know now, for instance, that vinyl chloride causes cancer—angiosarcomas of the liver. Twenty-three workers in vinyl-chloride plants, ravaged by liver cancer, have already died. Yet workers are still allowed to be exposed to it, breathing in reduced but potentially still harmful amounts of the substance that may very well lead to their eventual deaths. The Hiroshima studies show an increased incidence of all types of malignancies, but especially leukemia following exposures to nuclear radiation. There is some question today of there being no lower limit, no threshold, to the amounts of radiation associated with an increased risk of cancer. While experts argue as to the risks involved in exposures to the small amounts of radiation released in discharges during normal operations of nuclear power plants, there is no argument at all as to the risks involved following a nuclear accident. All experts agree that excluding those people killed immediately following the accident, an additional 40,000 to 100,000 more will eventually die from radiation-acquired cancers. And yet with other sources of energy available, men who should be guarding our health continue to allow nuclear-reactor plants to be built, potentially dooming, because of their ignorance or near-sightedness, other families and other toddlers.

Russia, West Germany and the World Health Association have all banned the use of Red Dye 2, a food coloring, because their studies of the dye, which is really a chemical, have shown it might cause cancer. Yet in the United States the men we should trust the most, those appointed to the Federal Drug Administration, have recently, for no better reason than to have our maraschino cherries redder, approved it for unlimited use. There will be no way to stay away from it, to keep it out of our bodies; it will be in lipsticks, pill coatings, liquid medicines, candy bars, non-cola soft drinks, gelatin desserts, baked goods, cakes and puddings, breakfast cereals, cold meats, frankfurters, sausages, vinegar, salad dressings, pretzels, canned fruit, sweet rolls and corn chips. Some researchers feel that any cancer produced by Red Dye 2 will be the kind with few antigens on their surface, the kind of cancer our immune system can least protect us against.

Cigarette smoking does produce that kind of low-antigen cancer. Three hundred thousand people will die of inoperable lung cancer in the next five years, maybe more, for no other reason than that they smoke, and the smoke they inhale produces cancer which their immune system cannot destroy. In an article in *Lancet,* the British medical journal, it was clearly put:

> Recent evidence [about lung cancer] allows the formation of a different hypothesis for the etiology of lung cancer in the smoker, which also includes a mechanism for the enhanced prevalence rate of repeated respiratory infection and subsequent chronic bronchitis associated with smoking. Firstly, the vapor phase of cigarette smoke (excluding tars and particulates) has been shown to be as effective in eliciting early tumor production in mice and changes in cell cultures as whole smoke. Secondly, cigarette smoke inhalation has been shown to affect deleteriously the immune response to both

human smokers and chronically exposed mice. Consequently, local immunity in the respiratory tract, which most certainly functions to protect the host from the development of infections and most probably the development of cancer, may be damaged by inhalation of cigarette smoke.

Despite all this evidence, we are still encouraged for the profit of the tobacco industry and its advertising agencies to continue smoking, while those we have entrusted with our safety and our health look the other way or issue token warnings. It is like Ibsen's play *An Enemy of the People,* in which the government in the interest of business and profit allows the tourists to use the typhoid-filled baths. Only now it is not fictional characters in a make-believe play we're dealing with, but ourselves and our children; it is not bacteria and viruses that are of concern, but cancer-causing poisons. We are now the tourists allowed and even encouraged to use, unknowing and uncomplaining, the deadly products—for no other reason than greed and profit.

17

Beyond Immunology

WE KNOW A GREAT DEAL today about the immune system, much that was not even dreamed of as little as twenty years ago, most of it discovered within the last five. Medically speaking, we are living today in the age of immunology. The great majority of articles in the leading medical journals, the most discussed topic at the great research symposiums, the main section of the specialty boards in both medicine and pediatrics, the overwhelming thrust of all contemporary medical research and concern, indeed of almost all modern medical thought, are immunological.

Yet for all its successes, despite its breakthroughs in treatment and diagnosis, the new insights immunology has given into both health and disease, there is the growing sense that we are no longer being that well served by it—that what has been accomplished in medicine and what is still being attempted cannot be all there is, that something terribly vital is missing. We know, even if no one tells us, that the whole man is greater than the sum of his parts, and there is a feeling we all have that in treating him only as a condition, as a heart attack or a kidney infection, as so much of this compound or that molecule, doctors have substituted the technology of medicine for—to use an almost forgotten term—its art, and science for its ability to heal.

It is indeed a fact that our heart does pump, our kidneys do filter, our immune system does protect. But it is also a fact that during the development of modern medical thought, in the midst of its ever newer and more startling discoveries, the whole man was at first put aside, then increasingly ignored, and finally discarded.

Galen began it back in the first century by telling us that the sense of grief we feel in our hearts when a friend dies, or the tenseness in our chest when we are frightened, is in reality of no significance, that the heart is simply a pump, nothing more. Later we were separated from that gripping, burning sensation in our stomachs by the scientists who assured us that the stomach is no more than a sack, a simple chemical dissolver of proteins, fats and sugars. James Gamble carried us further away from ourselves by defining the blood in terms of its salt and mineral concentrations; Herman by telling us that hearing is nothing but the oscillations of three small bones vibrating in our head. Our muscles became mere pulleys, fibers of the contractile protein actin, combining with myosin; our brains nothing more than a billion electrically discharging neurons. Through the years, medicine has been on a continual path of separation and isolation, the parts of men gradually becoming greater than man himself.

Not that the strength and astonishing effectiveness of that path can be denied. The worth of being able to say unequivocally that a sick child's potassium is 8.1 rather than 3.5, that this heart has a ventricular septal defect while that one has aortic stenosis, is as obvious for adequate diagnosis as it is necessary for definitive treatments. The ability this path has given medicine to give precise physical and chemical answers applicable to sick people collectively, no matter who or what they might be, is an amazing, unarguable achievement. It is a path that has turned medicine into a true lifesaving science, but springing as it does from the tradition of the scientific method, it has forced medicine to deal only with what can be measured, felt or seen. The force that has fueled all this is the same force that has fueled all the other sciences—technology: the development of those tools that enable us to look at our world and at ourselves in one particular, though effective way—physically. The union of medicine and technology has been incredibly productive, forging in its own crucible an ever more powerfully technical medical complex as sure of itself in the physical and chemical world as it is limited by it.

Ask a surgeon today on any kidney transplant service what he thinks of a psychiatrist coming onto his ward to help with the patients who are not doing well, to consult on those patients unable to go home because of acute tubular necrosis or infected shunts, to give some direction as to how to deal with the depressed adolescent girl rejecting her father's donated kidney, or the hostile patient undergoing his second rejection, and the surgeon will probably dismiss the idea. "If the kidney starts working," he will say, "they'll be okay. And besides," he might add, "we've got enough crazy people around here without adding another one."

Ask the neurologist what he thinks of the mind. "You mean the brain, don't you?" Complain to your physician that you are not feeling well, and he will give you an iron pill or a tranquilizer. "Take one before going to bed." Ask your gastroenterologist whether your ulcer might be from the terrible strain you are working under, and he will hand you some Maalox. "This will help; take one ounce three times daily between meals and before retiring." Mention to the professor of medicine that death is more frequent in families of bereaved relatives than families without grief, and he will simply shrug. "Dying of heartbreak? Unheard of." Ask the immunologist what he thinks of willing yourself to be ill, and he won't even answer.

Yet it has been known for decades that mice, after being in nothing more than a stressful environment, when placed in a tub of water will give up swimming and drown well before any unstressed mouse, and that rats crowded together will mysteriously absorb their fetuses rather than give birth. What about the woman who can lift a 3,000-pound car to save her trapped child? Or the patient who wants to die, or is convinced he is going to die, and does die, in spite of medical and surgical efforts that have regularly saved others with exactly the same physical condition?

Medicine might be able to ignore this other side of things, but we can't because we know, even if our surgeons and internists don't, that we are connected with our bodies, that the catch in our breath when we are startled, the tension in our guts when we're worried, the exhaustion we feel from our anxiety are as much a part of our illnesses as are the bacteria, viruses and auto-antibodies which attack us, and can in fact be just as debilitating and just as deadly. We know that a man coming home from a coronary care unit and labeled by his physician as cured of his heart attack, yet fearful of walking too fast or going on a plane, terrified of every increase in his heart rate, of the strain of sexual activity, can hardly be viewed by anyone, except maybe his doctor, as being healed of his illness. A recent Mayo Clinic study showed that 70 percent of all patients admitted to the Clinic had either a primary psychiatric diagnosis or a secondary psychiatric concern contributing substantially to their illness.

That illness may be psychological has long been a known, if begrudged, fact of medicine, yet the psychic origins of disease have been and still are almost totally ignored by medical science. As doctors, we keep prescribing pills, implanting pacemakers into hearts, cutting down amounts of salt in hypertension, making our patients watch calories for obesity, looking always at the physical part of disease, at those aspects of illness that can be attended to by our machines and our drugs: the sodiums, potassiums, cholesterol levels, the amounts of circulating renins, and angiotension.

As physicians we have always attempted to control diseases by conquering them. From ancient times, medicine has thought of disease as something from the outside, first as an attack by evil spirits, then as an attack by microbes and now as attacks by internal substances once normal but changed. Diseases were caused by insults from the outside, and so were to be handled from the outside. Drugs, surgery, machines became the arsenal of medicine, an armamentarium directed at attacking the attacker, at cutting it out, isolating it, killing it. This idea still continues to rule modern medical thought.

At a recent international medical meeting one of the foremost researchers in America felt compelled to warn his associates about the interpretation of skin testing for allergic conditions. He told of two supposedly severely allergic patients referred to him after being fully examined at two other large medical centers, during both of which previous hospitalization they had been negative for all skin tests. On admission to his hospital they were both completely worked up again in the hope of discovering this time what they were allergic to, but again all the applied skin tests were negative.

Depressed that after traveling thousands of miles expecting to be helped, or at least to have their allergy diagnosed, only to be told once more that nothing could be found and that they would have to go home again with no diagnosis and so no treatment, they began to complain bitterly to everyone around about the failure of medicine. They became so abusive to their young intern that in self-defense he said, half jokingly, that if only their skin tests would become positive, a diagnosis could be made, medications given, and they would be cured.

"The next morning," the researcher stated, "both patients had positive skin tests." His warning was lightly, if somewhat nervously, dismissed by the physicians present at the conference. There was no discussion; the implication of what he had said was completely ignored. People making their own skin tests positive? Impossible!

But doctors at the University of North Carolina, Chapel Hill, tell of the occasional patient sent to them from the back hills of the Carolinas and Georgia with a physical condition they are totally unable to diagnose, with fevers, aches and pains they cannot even begin to treat. Yet they have seen such patients totally cured when, sent home, they have had their own "root" doctors treat them with nothing more than the laying on of hands or the drinking of herbs. Even with the auto-immune diseases, the newest of the discovered causes of human illness, we still look for the outside agent—the virus or poison—which has somehow caused the change in normal tissue, leading to the production of auto-antibodies, and so to the disease.

BUT LIKE Fracastorius and Paracelsus, like Jenner and Metchnikoff, Koch, Halsted, Semmelweis and Pasteur, there are today, as there have always been in every generation, those few physicians who see that what has been accepted and what is practiced is no longer enough, that new theories must be proposed and new actions must be taken.

Today at a Southwestern medical center a specialist in the treatment of cancer, himself a victim of ulcer disease and like any layman forced to take antacids to relieve his pain, small feedings, milk and atropine to cut down his gastric acidity, came to sense that the fault for his illness might be *his* rather than his stomach's, that his suffering was something he might be responsible for, something he might be doing or not doing to himself. He wondered, too, about other diseases, about other patients' responsibility for their own illnesses, and in the early seventies he started on a daring, unheard-of experiment. He began to have some of his cancer patients, in addition to their regular medical treatments, meditate on their tumors, try to heal themselves.

He continues to treat his cancer patients with the conventional radiotherapy, the cobalt machines and the antimetabolic drugs used for cancer sufferers all over the world. But he also tells them about their bodies. He explains what their antibodies are, what the molecules look like, where they are made. He tells them about their cancers, about how the antibodies are molded to couple with the antigens on the surface of their tumor cells. He tells them about their immune system, how it originally had gone after their first tumor cells, trying to destroy them before they could get a foothold, how the complement circulating in their bloodstream was activated by the coupling of antibodies with these newly formed tumor cells. He tells them about their white cells, their T and B lymphocytes, about the messenger lymphocytes in their circulation; the tranformation to killer cells. He tell them about how it all works and how in their particular case their immune system, despite all its efforts, had been beaten back and then overwhelmed by their cancer cells.

He explains what the radiation therapy is supposed to do, how the rads from the cobalt machine and the anticancer drugs will kill some tumor cells and weaken others, how the killing will release cancer antigens into their bloodstream, flooding their immune system, stimulating the production of more anticancer antibodies and more killer lymphocytes so that their immune system can again begin its attack.

He tells his patients how their white cells and macrophages will flood in over the radiated tumor, work their way down into the irradiated, drug-filled malignant mass and begin to devour the cancer cells, not only those sickened or dying from the radiation and the ingested antimetabolites but the ones unaffected, too. He shows them their X-rays with the masses in their stomachs or in their chest so they will know what they are up against. He describes their circulation to them, where their arteries are and their veins, just how their blood will bring their newly formed antibodies and white cells to and from their tumors. He makes sure his patients grasp the anatomy of their disease, that they know exactly how their antibodies, T and B lymphocytes, complement, granulocytes and macrophages will make the fight.

When they understand their disease and the avenues over which their cure could come, when they know how healing can be effected, the physician begins to teach them to meditate—not on spiritual concerns, nor on their wish for comfort, relief, tranquillity or acceptance—but on themselves. He has them visualize their tumors, the wildly growing cancer cells within their otherwise healthy bodies, and then he has them do something that has never been done in medicine before—he has them meditate on the battle between themselves and their disease. He tells them to turn inward, to think of their antibodies, to consciously try to will them toward their tumors, to make their killer lymphocytes take up a more vigorous attack against their cancer cells, more of their macrophages to take part in the battle. He has them conjure up their own internal defenses, to do what we never think of doing, what we have been taught to leave not just to others, but to nobody—the defense of ourselves, the bending of our own minds to the task of our own personal survival.

Very few physicians are really comfortable with what this doctor is doing; but since his cases are so hopeless, since his associates know so little can be done, anyway, and since his efforts do include the normally accepted medical treatments for cancer patients, he is left alone. If anything, he is bemusedly tolerated.

There are other researchers trying to do similar things, working in other areas of medicine, who are not so gently treated. Understaffed and underpaid, overworked and ridiculed, they continue nonetheless to devote their time and energies to the new idea that people can be made responsible for their own health, for their own cures. These are the researchers who are now out at the borders of medical thought, trying against much resistance and the usual age-old prejudices to close the last great gap in medicine, the distance that has grown between our diseases and ourselves.

"I'm Dr. Scheel," the researcher says to the student who is cooperating in the experiment. "I want to make sure you understand what we're trying to do, what this experiment is all about. Don't let all this equipment bother you. It's really very simple, but I'm sure as you'll realize before we finish, quite important, potentially crucial not only for a real understanding of how disease happens but even more important, an understanding of the part we can play in supporting our own health."

They are sitting in the basement of the psychology building —in a room which has been partitioned off from the furnace and storage areas.

"As you know, this is an experiment that will test the ability of human beings to voluntarily control their own skin temperature. Usually skin temperature is under involuntary control, apparently changing without any conscious thought, going up or down in response only to whether our body needs to maintain or lose heat. In short, what is involved is a response where the body seems to take care of itself without any help from us. But we believe people can, by thinking, voluntarily control their temperature, make their skin hotter or colder as they wish, that they can consciously master what before seemed beyond their control. For this experiment, though, we will be concerned only with the skin temperature of our fingers—index fingers, to be exact. But remember, what happens to the skin of our fingers should be applicable to skin anywhere else.

"The cubicle you see there in front of you, behind the one-way mirror, is a temperature control room that will be heated at a constant temperature; it's also fairly soundproof. That's where the experiment will be conducted. During the experiment you'll be lying on the bed you can see from here. I'll be able from out here to keep an eye on you in case anything goes wrong. We can communicate with each other through the speaker system you see in front of you and the squawk box there on the inside wall of the cubicle. Now let me tell you about the experiment itself.

"Two thermistors, tiny electrodes, will be placed on the skin at the bottom of your left and right index fingers—the soft fleshy part directly under the nail. These thermistors are the means of measuring the temperature in your fingers. As the temperature changes, they transmit the changes as electrical signals. I'll monitor the signals out here. You'll be wearing a set of earphones that will allow you to monitor these signals too. While I'm watching you I'll be making sure throughout the experiment, in a sense monitoring you, to see you are relaxed and don't unknowingly clench your fist which would, of course, raise the temperature in your fingers. Okay, let's go in and I'll show you how the whole thing works."

"Those temperature devices, the thermistors," the student asks, "they aren't going to be stuck into my fingers, are they?"

"No, they're just pasted on. There'll be no sticking you with anything, no injections, no pain." Scheel opens the door and follows the student into the cubicle.

He picks up the two electrodes. "These are the thermistors. The wires that come out of them run into the floor and from there to a sound amplifier, then to my control board as well as into your earphones. Why don't you lie down and I'll show you?

"The temperature of your skin will be measured by the thermistors and then amplified into sound. The earphones will allow you to tell when the temperature in one finger exceeds the temperature in the other. When both fingers are at the same temperature, you will hear an equal tone that will appear from the earphones to be coming from the center of your head. When the temperature in, say, your left finger goes up compared to your right finger, the sound you will be hearing through the earphone will go up in tone and seem to move to the left. This will indicate that the temperature in your left finger is higher than the temperature in your right. Again, the sound you will be hearing is dependent only on the temperatures in your two fingers, the fingers to which the thermistors are attached. Now I think it's probably best for you to put on the earphones and see how they feel. I'll help you."

When the ear set is in place, Scheel connects the thermistors. "I'll be recording the changes in temperature on a permanent record. Now I'll go outside to start the recording equipment, and to make sure everything is functioning properly."

The student looks at him apprehensively.

"Oh, don't worry. There are no shocks involved with this. You won't feel a thing. The only thing that you'll hear is the tone through the earphones, that's all."

Back in the control room, Scheel switches on the amplifier. There is a hum and then a pure tone comes out of the speaker over his head. He flicks on the recording device, and turning up the amplifier, talks into the microphone.

"That sound you're hearing is the sound generated by the thermistors recording the temperature in each of your two fingers. What I want you to do, and I will say this three times, is to make your left finger warm and your right finger cold. Now we'll begin, but gradually. Make your left arm warm and your right arm cold. Make your left hand warm and your right hand cold. Make your left index finger warm, make your right index finger cold . . . Now again, make your left arm warm . . ." He repeats the instructions a second time and a third. "Now," he adds slowly, "what I want you to do when the sound changes is to think that thought again, whatever that thought was—the thought right before you heard the sound change—think that thought again. All right, let's try it once more. Make your left arm warm and your right arm cold . . ."

Scheel remembers his first patient, that same look of confusion, the same struggle to understand what was expected of him, much less how to do it.

"Now make your left arm warm, your right arm cold. Just relax," he says soothingly. "We have lots of time . . . Now make your left hand warm, your right hand cold."

Forty-five minutes later Scheel stops the session, walks into the cubicle and takes the earphones off the student. "Don't worry. It takes a while, but it will work . . . Same time tomorrow."

Halfway through the next session, the tone suddenly changes. The stylus on the recorder moves up and to the left. Scheel looks through the one-way mirror at the subject, who also has heard the tone change and looks pleased with himself.

"Good," Scheel says into the microphone. "Now think that

same thought again, whatever it was, the same thought . . . Now make your left finger warm and your right finger cold."

Some subjects have told Scheel they tried to think of warmth traveling down their left hand; others said they thought, without doing it, of clenching their fist, while still others pretended their right hand was suddenly dunked into ice water; some even thought of the excitement of sexual activity, of using their left hand to stroke a girl's body; others thought of fear.

"I guess I just thought of my arm relaxing and being warm," the subject volunteers after the session. "And then the tone changed, and I knew I'd done it; I could even feel my finger suddenly get warm."

By the seventh session the subject can maintain a temperature difference of one degree between his two index fingers; by the tenth, a constant two-degree difference. More important to Scheel, by the fourteenth session the subject can alternate the temperature changes back and forth almost instantaneously.

"I can do it anywhere now," the student says at the end of the final session. "Even without the earphones. I don't even have to think about it. I just do it. I might not even need gloves this winter," he adds jokingly. "At least on my index fingers."

But Scheel doesn't laugh. He knows of those patients suffering from a disease called Raynaud's phenomenon, where cold makes these people's fingers blanch and then painfully ulcerate. In cold weather they have to wear gloves. Maybe, he thinks, just maybe . . .

BUT THIS WORK is not only happening with abilities as crude as temperature control. In other experiments at another medical center, microelectrodes have been attached to the tiny nerves in a subject's arm going to a single one of his muscle groups. The subject, seeing the discharges of his own nerve cell portrayed on an electronic screen, establishes a connection with his inner self, a way of controlling what before would have been considered beyond anyone's conscious control. Using the impulses on the screen rather than sound, he learns eventually how to locate and control that single muscle group hidden away in the muscle mass of his arm. Later, even without the screen, he can identify this microscopic group of cells, unviewable to him and unsensed, barely able to be located by the researcher himself, only one group of cells out of the subject's hundreds of trillions, and yet he can, after ten hourly sessions, consciously single out that cell group from all the rest of the cells in his body and make it jump or lie still, dance or rest as he wishes.

This kind of work is ignored, dismissed patronizingly by the medical establishment as essentially unimportant, and even if interesting, still a worthless accomplishment. But these new researchers have proceeded with their work. They have widened the cracks that first appeared in the thirties in medicine's long-established dogmas that diseases are external in origin and therefore treatment should be directed against the external threats, that we are unable to heal ourselves because we are not responsible for our illnesses. The dogma sustains itself on the belief that with the development of ever more effective drugs, better machines and more radical surgery will come ever more dramatic cures.

In those early thirties, a paper was published in the *Journal of the American Medical Association* by a physician who had evaluated thirty-five different published studies on the use of drugs in the treatment of high blood pressure. The author found to his surprise that every paper he'd looked at boasted either complete or significant partial relief from the material being tested. These papers variously claimed that mistletoe, diathermy, watermelon extract, even drops of dilute hydrochloric acid three times a day brought improvement in over 85 percent of the patients.

Since all the substances tested were so radically different chemically one from the other, the author was forced to conclude that the only thing all the studies had in common was that "the patients wanted to improve, they wanted their doctors to be successful, they wanted the drugs to work, they wanted to get better." He attributed the successes in the studies to the well-known but little discussed "placebo effect."

A placebo is a drug that isn't a drug. It is a pill, a compound, an additive or a liquid given to a patient by a physician with no expectation that it will have any therapeutic effect whatever.

A small scientific wedge had been driven into the accepted

medical concept that diseases as well as successful treatments must all be physical, but apparently the paper went unnoticed at the time. Fifteen years later Dubos, the famous biologist, widened that wedge by writing honestly for the first time what no one would admit. "Although placebos are scarcely mentioned in the medical literature, they are administered more than any other group of drugs. . . . Few doctors admit they give placebos, yet there is a placebo ingredient in practically every prescription. . . . The placebo is a potent agent and its action can resemble almost any drug."

Every doctor agrees, whether he likes it or not, that the odor of tincture of benzoin makes the inhalation of steam much more acceptable and therapeutic to his ill patients than the inhalation of steam itself, even though he knows there is no scientific reason for his patients' feeling better, or for their conviction that they are helped more from the benzoin-treated mixture than if he had just prescribed the steam alone.

Placebos are given today as they have always been—although now it is not so unknowingly. They are given today when the doctor feels frustrated, or hostile, too busy to do anything else, or more likely when his patient is demanding and the doctor feels there is nothing further he can do but that he must do something. It has become the great secret of modern medicine. Physicians do not like to admit they've prescribed a compound they know could not possibly be effective. They feel guilty about it, and defensive. In the modern climate of laboratory-based medicine, it is threatening to them to admit they have to sink to what they consider charlatanism. They fear the loss of self-esteem and prestige among their colleagues if they are found out, and the loss of respect from their patients. They also feel threatened and vulnerable in having to order placebos, in having to give up what they consider to be the scientifically sound therapeutic methods of medicine. They have learned to hide behind this therapeutic shield not only from themselves but from their patients' real fears, withdrawing from the practice of the more difficult and lonely art of medicine by prescribing medications they know or have been told should work, without their having to get involved.

But the placebos they are forced to use are effective; they relieve, they comfort, and for a time, for some people, they even appear to heal when all of modern medical science has failed or when, because of the desperateness or uniqueness of the disease, medicine even with its great achievements offers no hope of success. Modern medical science is simply unable to explain the "placebo effect." It has no theories on which even to begin. Yet those empty pills, those sugared waters, work now as they always have.

IT TOOK two extraordinary events in the practice of clinical medicine for those who pondered the relationship of health and disease, as well as the effectiveness of placebos, to begin to chart a course which could bring medicine back to the realization that its province is internal as well as external.

The first began some twenty years ago, when a physician had his patients learn to control their own heartbeats by following a timer, just as later subjects would use headsets and oscilloscopes to control temperatures and muscle cells. He had his patients listen to their heart as they watched the timer. If they failed to increase their heart rate by the amount wanted within the proper time, they received a shock. By the third hourly session these subjects could, by concentrating their attention on the timer, control their own heart rate, speeding it up enough to avoid the shock before the timer triggered the current. But when this happened it was the time of the beginnings of transplants, of kidney biopsies, of dialysis, antibody isolation, the discovery of complement activation, the Sabin polio vaccine, the conquering of Rh incompatibility, and the first understandings of the auto-immune diseases. For almost two decades, overshadowed by the new discoveries of immunology and overwhelmed by the new operative techniques of both medicine and surgery, the amazing discovery that people could at will speed up their own heartbeats was ignored.

The second event occurred some years later, in 1969, with the publication in the prestigious *Annals of Internal Medicine* of an article titled "The Relationship of Premature Ventricular Contractions (PVC) to Coronary Heart Disease and Sudden Death in the Tecumseh Epidemiological Study." With scientific stiffness the article stated what physicians had felt for over half a century—that the occurrence of premature ventricular contractions, a rather common type of arrhythmia found in many cardiac patients, was associated with an increased incidence of sudden death.

The article stated that the diagnosis of PVC's in patients with cardiac disease was in essence a potential death sentence —and those with the PVC's did die, some while walking to their cars, others raking the lawn, many just sitting talking or even lying in bed. Faced with the unarguable scientific evidence that this type of arrhythmia was potentially dangerous, physicians were driven to giving these patients potent cardiac drugs: digitalis, propanalol, atropine, edrophonium, phenylephrine, phentolamine—drugs to stabilize the heart in the hope of stopping or holding in check the PVC's before they went on to cause a heart attack. But the drugs, all of them, had their own drawbacks; and most, even if pushed to toxicity, still didn't work all that well or caused dangerous arrhythmias themselves.

At the time this article appeared, experimental animal studies were being conducted on the physiology of the heart. These studies showed that the nerves going to the heart could, by being stimulated mechanically, affect the heart's rate of contraction. By changing that rate, dramatic decreases in the number and duration of experimentally induced PVC's could be produced. The foundation of a new kind of medicine was set. It took only the insight and courage of the new group of medical researchers, aware of the new developments in internal control, to begin to find a better way to treat these PVC patients.

In the early nineteen-seventies two doctors, one in the department of psychiatry at the University of Pennsylvania, the other in the department of medicine, faced with cardiac patients suffering from PVC's, wondered if those heart nerves that had been stimulated mechanically in the experimental animal studies could not be put under their patients' conscious control and give the same results. Might not people, like the patients in the heart-timer experiments, be able to put their own heart rate under voluntary control, speeding it up or slowing it down at will, stopping their own PVC's?

The initial experiment used only eight patients, but it was enough to mark the beginning of a new therapeutic age. The researchers' experiment, as reported, makes extraordinary reading. Even a summary of their original report shows the simple eloquence of their method, the indisputable proof of what was accomplished and what might yet be done in other areas of medicine.

Selection. The eight patients with PVC's (Premature Ventricular Contractions) were selected from Baltimore City Hospitals, and from referrals by private physicians. Each patient was told in detail about the nature of the experiment, and he was allowed to inspect all his data throughout the study.

Hospitalization procedure. Patients were hospitalized for the duration of the study and given passes each weekend. After admission, they were given a complete physical examination and a standard battery of laboratory tests including a 12 lead electrocardiogram and X-rays.

Experimental Design–Biofeedback

Laboratory. During the study, the patient lay in a hospital bed in a sound-deadened room. At the foot of the bed was a vertical display of three differently colored light bulbs, an intercom and a meter.

The three lights provided the patient with feedback information about his cardiac function. The top light (green) and the bottom light (red) were cue lights. The middle light (yellow) was the reinforcer; it was on when the patient was producing the correct heart-rate response.

One to three 80-minute conditioning sessions were carried out daily. A typical session began with about 10 minutes for the attaching of electrocardiogram leads, and a strain gauge around the lower chest to monitor breathing.

During the initial or control session, the patient simply lay in bed in the laboratory for the prescribed time period. The feedback lights were never turned on. Next, heart-rate speeding was taught for about ten sessions. For about ten further sessions, the patient alternately had to increase and decrease his heart rate during the periods of one to four minutes throughout the session. During these sessions, the green and red cue lights would come on alternately so that the patient would know whether to speed up or to slow down his heart rate.

In the last training session the patient had to maintain his heart rate between pre-set upper and lower limits. Only the yellow light would be on when the heart rate was within this range. When the rate was too fast, the yellow light would go off, and the red light would go on, cueing the patient to slow down. When the rate was too slow, the green light would come on, cueing the patient to speed up. These training sessions also gave the patient feedback every time he had a premature ventricular contraction.

Initially, the feedback was available for one minute and unavailable for three; in the final sessions, it was on for one minute and off for seven. By this procedure, the patient was weaned from the light feedback and made to become aware of his PVC's through his own sensations.

Follow-up. Clinical follow-up was done in the Hospital's Cardiac Clinic and by the referring physicians. The visits usually included electrocardiograms with a one-half minute rhythm strip.

The small number of subjects used exposed the study to the ridicule that medical science has been using for over a hundred years to flay experiments that do not fit its bias. "What were the controls?" "Where are the statistics?" "How do you know the patients didn't get better because of something else?" "Statistically the mathematics don't hold up." "Did they really control all the variables?" "How do you know that drugs aren't just as good?" "Pacemakers work just as well." "What we have already is good enough if used right."

But the results could not be totally ignored. In the original article the researchers went on in the discussion section to report their results with scientific restraint but still in the human terms that have always given medicine its real worth:

Patient 1. LR, a 52-year-old Caucasian female, had a history of five myocardial infarctions in the thirteen years prior to study. In association with the last two, eight months and five months prior to study, she had premature ventricular contractions. Maintenance quinidine therapy was required to suppress [the arrhythmias] after the last myocardial infarction. She had been on digoxin for one year. Because of persistent diarrhea (from the medication) the quinidine was discontinued two weeks prior to the study, and premature ventricular contractions increased in frequency from one to two per minute to ten per minute. . . .

During the sessions, the patient consistently maintained

her heart rate with the predetermined low beat range (usually 60–70 beats/min.) and premature ventricular contractions were infrequent.

After a three-week recess, the patient's digoxin was stopped. The only discernible effect was an increase in baseline heart rate of about five beats/min. to about 68. Twenty-three further sessions were carried out. Gradually the patient's feedback was decreased (and without the further use of any monitoring devices) her premature ventricular contractions remained very low. She was discharged off all medications.

Not all the eight patients in the study were helped; some had hearts too damaged for anything to work, for some it was too late, but for the others it was enough. They had learned to control their own PVC's. Like the first patient, they were discharged, a few off all medication, free of drugs for the first time in years, no longer forced each day to take their pills, no longer troubled by their drug-induced diarrheas. They had become responsible for their own health.

The results of this experiment were published over four years ago, yet even today there remains a reluctance among physicians to accept not only the facts of the study but the implications: a new type of therapy, a new way to look at disease. As before, the present is sacrificed to the past and everyone suffers for it; prejudiced and nonprejudiced alike become casualties of dogma and bias. Before Pasteur, the son of the physician fighting the use of the rabies vaccine as unnatural died just as quickly if bit by a rabid dog and just as grotesquely as any grocer's boy; the farmer dying of smallpox in Jenner's time could just as well have been the surgeon who argued against the immorality of vaccination. Today the ulcer patient taking his Maalox to stop his stomach pains might just as well be the professor of internal medicine prescribing his own Maalox. All pay the price.

THE IDEA of getting in touch with our inner selves, of becoming involved with our own disease, is growing. Other physicians responsible for caring for patients whose diseases seemed to be the result of their having lost some type of internal control have tried, when all of medicine's special skills and newly won

[243]

achievements offered no help, as the cardiac researchers did, the concept of biofeedback.

In the last three years, pediatric neurologists have used it with their seemingly hopeless patients—children born with open spines, with the nerves to the lower part of their bodies mutilated and nonfunctioning. These desperate children, born with congenitally defected spinal cords causing not only paralysis of their legs but uncontrollable bowels, have always been psychologically brutalized. Shy, withdrawn, they are unable to sit in a schoolroom for fear of being ridiculed for having to wear diapers, or terrified to stay overnight at a friend's house lest they soil themselves. Medicine's answer to their problem has been ineffective stool hardeners or colostomy bags. Then a few physicians tried biofeedback techniques and were able to write:

> Most children had been unable to control their stools for periods of four to eight years. By watching the pens on a polygraph both the patient and the therapist were provided precise feedback on the responses of the patient's internal and external sphincters to the stimulus of the inflation of a balloon placed in their rectums. In a few two-hour sessions the patients were able to learn the correct [internal] responses that enabled them to remain continent [have bowel control] for as long as they have been followed, from one and a half to five years.

With no effective medication available and no really appropriate surgery, modern medicine with all its great achievements was not enough. Yet these children could still be helped, by being taught to help themselves.

People with high blood pressure, too, have been able to learn to take care of themselves. British physicians using these same techniques of biofeedback have been able to teach hypertensive patients, some of whom have been on blood-pressure medications most of their adult life, to consciously lower their own blood pressure, to decrease their own reliance on medications—in short, to heal themselves.

But what about the rest of us? Sir William Osler, one of the greatest physicians of the late nineteenth century, is reputed to have said that to predict the outcome of tuberculosis—a common infectious disease in which a vigorous attack by the patient's immune system is critical to his survival—one must know what is going on in the patient's head.

Almost seventy-five years later, in 1951, Dr. Day, a British authority studying tuberculosis patients, wrote along these same lines: "To develop chronic active tuberculosis a person needs some bacteria, lungs, and some internal or external factor which lowers the resistance to the disease." Day went on to state that unhappiness is—not can be, but is—a cause of such lowered resistance.

Families of ill children are found to have been more disorganized during the six-month period before they became ill, and to have exposed their children to a greater number of disruptive psychological and social changes than did the families of a control group of healthy children. Prolonged recovery from influenza has also been linked with depression. A review of patients with rheumatoid arthritis indicates that patients who did poorly were more anxious and depressed than those with less severe, more easily handled disease.

It is not only medical diseases that seem to be affected by how we feel, but surgical diseases as well. And not only rare surgical diseases, but one of the most common affecting women today. Breast cancer was described by the ancient Egyptian surgeon Imhotep and yet even now, some five thousand years later, the best therapy is still in doubt. With one out of every fourteen women being operated on for this disease, no one knows yet which operation is best.

Radical mastectomy, which has been the most commonly performed operative procedure, is a brutal operation entailing the removal of not only the entire breast but all the underlying muscles and surrounding lymph nodes, even those going up to the arm. In 1964 Kaal and Johansen, comparing the results of radical and simple surgery (which involves only removal of the cancerous lump but otherwise leaves the breast intact), found no difference in survival. In 1969 Rissonen, in a trial of biopsy incision versus radical mastectomy, came to the same conclusion. On the other hand, in 1972 Atkins compared the simple removal of the lump with radical surgery, both plus radiotherapy, and claimed some superiority for the latter. In truth, the radical approach has never been compared in a satisfactory trial with the less mutilating conservative surgery, let alone an untreated group. Based on "common sense," the radical treatment is without scientific validation.

In a recent article in the *Journal of the Irish Medical Association* titled "Breast Cancer—Mistaken Concepts, Therapeutic Consequences and Future Implications," Edelstyn and Mac-Rae state that the radical removal of a woman's breast "might be defensible if there was no negative side to the treatment." In giving the negative reasons, the authors do not restrict their comments to the stiff shoulders and swollen arms, the bony chest wall and the crippling muscular atrophy resulting from the radical procedure, but go on to mention the mental stress of the disfiguring operation. They state: "Mental stress accompanying hospital attendance, and the socio-sexual implications of breast loss, unpleasant enough in itself, additionally carries the possibility . . . that [emotional stress and the anxiety of being disfigured] may contribute to immunosuppression [of the patient's defenses] . . . and that such immunosuppression could in itself lead to a heightened incidence of distant metastases [the spread of the original cancer to other organs] and death."

Anxiety leading to the spread of cancer is a new and important thought in regard to patient survival.

BUT ALL THIS WORK showing the connections between our minds and our bodies, all the new ideas and theories about our ability to heal ourselves would be scientifically meaningless if such connections could not be identified, if the physical interaction between the mind and the organs that protect us could not be proved.

In the early nineteen-sixties, direct proofs were established of the connection between the brain, where we do our thinking, and the rest of the body. Fessel demonstrated that mental stress alone produces a rise in a person's circulating Immunoglobulin M. Other researchers, working on animal brains, showed that destroying a small part of the brain in the area associated in humans with emotions would lead to a complete halt in the animals' antibody response, with the prolonged retention of antigens in these brain-damaged animals' bloodstream. Destruction of the same area in other experimental animals eliminated these animals' ability to reject any transplanted skin, while electronic stimulation rather than destruction of the area caused the direct opposite—a marked increase in the animal's ability to make antibodies, to respond to any injected antigen. Additional work on guinea pigs has shown that destruction of other parts of the brain not only protects the animals against certain forms of serum sickness but will decrease any kind of delayed hypersensitivity.

We are connected to our bodies. Engel, in a study of ulcerative colitis, a disease now known to be associated with auto-antibodies produced against the patient's own large bowel, found these patients to be obsessive, compulsive people anally oriented, indecisive, rigid and given to worrying. McClary, an Australian researcher, found that the onset of systemic lupus eyrthematosus often followed a major life-stress situation.

How we feel does affect functions that have long been considered to be beyond our thoughts or emotions. An increase in the severity of experimentally induced immune arthritis has been found in stressed rats when compared to control non-stressed rats. Electroshock stress administered three days prior to inoculation with a cancer-causing virus reduces the incidence and size of the tumors in the stressed animals, while such shocks administered three days following inoculation with the virus increases the size of the tumor.

We know, too, that the hormones we all have circulating in our blood are increased or decreased in amounts depending on how we feel, and that these hormones at times are released in staggering amounts: not only can adrenalin, corticosteroid, histamine, serotinin, kallikrein allow us to lift objects ten, twenty and thirty times our own weight, make our hearts race until we feel faint, kill us if we wish or send us to bed exhausted, but they have also been shown to individually and specifically affect all of the three different cell types of our immune system. Released by how we feel they regulate the movements and functioning of our macrophages and our killer T cells, as well as the antibody-producing abilities of our B lymphocytes.

The idea of the conscious control of our immune system does not seem so far-fetched any more. To use our minds to will our white cells into a more efficient attack against our infections, to voluntarily stop transplant rejections, does not now really seem so bizarre a notion.

There are a growing number of facts available that show

plainly we are as much a part of our own diseases as we are of our health, that we should be able to and indeed can help ourselves. The task of the physician today is what it has always been, to help the body do what it has learned so well to do on its own during its unending struggle for survival—to heal itself. To accomplish this we must remember what doctors have always had to remember, to "look and observe, go back to the bedside, be suspicious of eloquence, ignore ceremony." It is the body, not medicine, that is the hero.

About the Author

RONALD J. GLASSER, M.D., was born in Chicago, Illinois, and graduated from Johns Hopkins Medical School in 1965. He was intern and resident in pediatrics at the University of Minnesota Medical school (1965–68) and passed his specialist board in pediatrics while serving as major in the U.S. Army Medical Corps stationed in Japan. Returning to Minneapolis in 1970, he was on the staff of the Hennepin County General Hospital and an assistant professor in the Department of Pediatrics at the University of Minnesota Hospitals. The following year he began a National Institutes of Health Research Fellowship in pediatric kidney disease. At present he is an instructor in the Department of Pediatric Nephrology at the University of Minnesota Hospitals and lives in Minneapolis.

Dr. Glasser is the author of two widely praised books, *365 Days*, published in 1971, an account of a tour of duty treating soldiers in Vietnam, which won the *Washington Monthly* Political Book Award and was translated into eight languages, and the world-wide best-selling novel *Ward 402*, published in 1973. In addition, his writing has appeared in magazines and newspapers all over the country, including the *Atlantic, Harper's* and *Washington Monthly*.